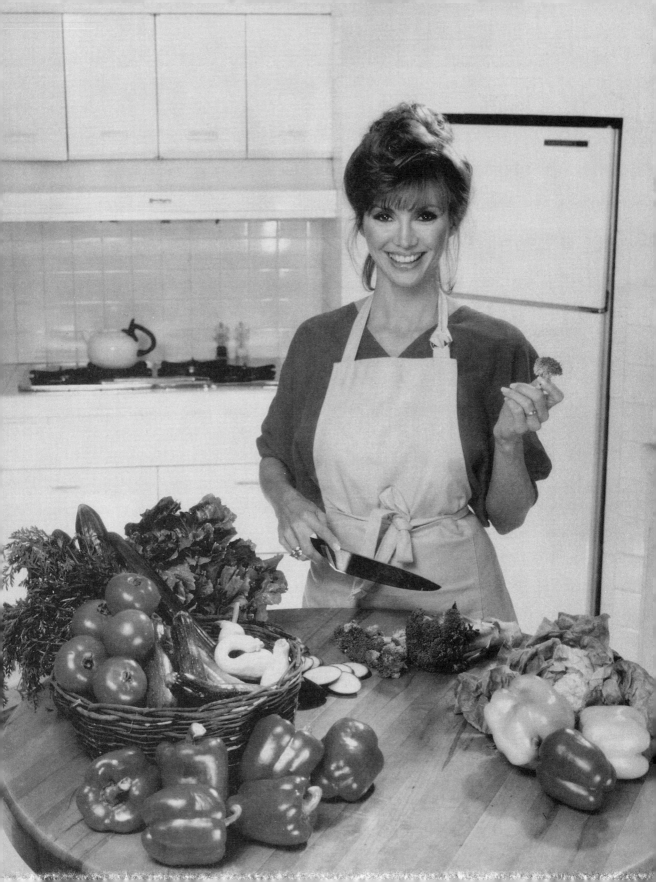

THE DIET PRINCIPAL

Victoria Principal

SIMON AND SCHUSTER New York

Also by Victoria Principal

The Body Principal
The Beauty Principal

```
┌─────────────────────────────────────────┐
│                                         │
│         FOR ANNIE . . .                 │
│         THROUGH THICK AND THIN          │
│                                         │
└─────────────────────────────────────────┘
```

ACKNOWLEDGMENTS

There are numerous people I would like to thank for their contributions to this book:

Dan Green for his masterly advice. Hermien Lee for so generously sharing her knowledge of nutrition. Dr. Bruce Gordon for his insight and his understanding of eating disorders. The senior staff at the Department of Health and Human Services in Washington, D.C., especially at the Food and Drug Administration. Jose Eber (for doing more than my hair!). Marja Webster. Jeremy Mariage. Janet Surmi. Donna Skrzypek. Mitchell Frieder. Chris Matsumoto and Flower Fashions...and for all the lovely pictures, Harry Langdon, Greg Gorman, Gary Bernstein, and Ronnie Kaufman.

CONTENTS

INTRODUCTION

Today is the first day of the rest of your thin life. Today is the last day of old, useless diets. I don't know how you got this book—whether you are browsing at this moment in a book store, whether it was a gift, or whether you purposefully chose it yourself. No matter how you got it, if you've read this far you're already on the way to a new, a better, a thinner life.

I can promise you that in your hands you are holding the diet that can truly change your life. After reading this book and learning and practicing the "Diet for Life," you will indeed have found the way to a life free of that terrible, hopelessly overwhelming "Fear of Fat"! No more malnutritious crash diets; no more binges and personal recriminations; no more promises to God (that you always break!); and no more feeling out of control.

Congratulations! You are about to enter a new phase of your life, one that is going to last *the rest* of your life. You are finally going to be healthy, thin, and, I hope, very happy. I sense your heart beating a little faster. You're trying not to acknowledge how excited and hopeful you are, afraid to believe that this is finally the diet that will help you, that this is really the answer you've been looking for, maybe for years. But you have found it. It's okay to smile—go ahead, smile really big because you are the person who is going to make this happen.

I'm supplying you with the blueprint—that has worked for me and countless others—for a long, healthy, and thin life. But it's *you* who is going to follow it; it's *you* who is going to make it happen; and it's *you* who is going to reap all the benefits.

So dance a jig, smile, even laugh—happy days are here again! You have just begun the first hour of the first day of your new, thin life.

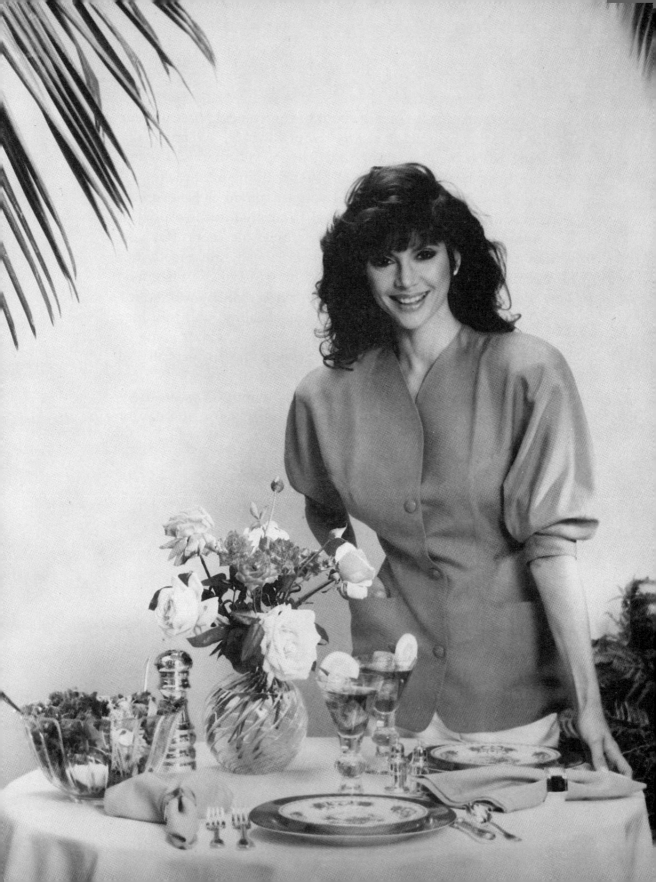

CHAPTER 1

THE DIET PRINCIPLES

When the phone rang that morning, I jumped. It wasn't that it was so early—I had in fact been up for some time, had already taken a short walk along the beach, and had eaten my rather substantial breakfast. It was just that the phone hadn't rung that much lately. I had been living at the beach for several months, trying to put some distance between myself and Hollywood. I had reached a point in my professional life where I was so disappointed with the parts I was being offered that I had decided to slow down the pace of my life and wait for the role that would let me show the kind of work I was capable of doing.

The good scripts weren't plentiful. I found myself leading a very quiet life, spending a lot of time by myself, thinking, resting, trying to shake the tension that had been building up the last few years, and waiting for the phone to bring me the good news.

Thus when the phone rang that morning, I jumped. My agent excitedly gave me the news. There was a good role in a new movie, and both the writer and director wanted to talk to me about it. My agent would send the script over immediately.

It arrived at noon. I finished reading it at four. He was right —it was a great role. I was ecstatic—finally I would be taken seriously. I could return to acting, to the life I loved.

I remember going upstairs to call my agent, eager to tell him how much I loved the script and how excited I was about doing the part. On the way to the phone I passed the full-length mirror that hung on my closet door. I stopped to look, and suddenly I knew that I could not accept the part. I couldn't even go to meet the director or the writer. I couldn't meet anyone; I couldn't even think of returning to the public eye because I was nearly 40 pounds overweight.

Anyone can gain weight. It doesn't happen only to the rich or poor, or only to brunettes, redheads, or blonds. Anyone can eat too much occasionally or regularly. Anyone can become someone they don't want to be. It happens for many reasons—depression, unhappiness, feelings of insecurity, or just plain letting yourself go. But it had never happened to me, and I was scared.

I was also heartbroken. And, frankly, ashamed. It seemed to me to have happened overnight, and I couldn't figure out how it had happened without my knowledge. Six months before, I had the body I had always been proud of; now I had a body I only wanted to hide. It seemed to me that the weight had sort of sneaked up on me—one day I was slim and fit, and the next I was fat.

But of course that was not what had happened. The realization that I was gaining weight had come a little bit every day, but like most people, I chose to ignore the signs. If I had been honest with myself every time I looked in the mirror, I would have seen the extra eight pounds, then ten pounds, then twelve. But I always figured that if I wanted to, I would just take off the extra weight.

And suddenly, it was 40 pounds. Forty pounds is a lot for anyone to gain, but on my very small build it was an enormous amount—I had ballooned from 105 to over 140, and it seemed disastrous to me.

Once I began to think about how it had happened, it wasn't too difficult to figure out. I had "retired" from my hectic and tense life, convinced that I had to take a sabbatical to avoid becoming another Hollywood casualty. I moved to the beach, removed myself from the social whirl, isolated myself from business associates and friends, and waited for the better parts to come. There were offers, but they weren't the kind I wanted and I was determined to stick it out. I was convinced that the next part would be the right one, the one that would be offered to me for my acting ability and not the "sexiness" of my looks. So I waited. I was somewhat depressed, frequently alone, and one of the few pleasures I had was eating. For the first time in my life, I found myself taking solace in food.

I realized that little by little I had let food become my tranquilizer. Unconsciously I had resumed doing what I had done as a teenager, which was eating four meals a day (then it had never showed on my body; now it added up). I began eating meat, which I had not done in years. I prepared large, lavish meals that involved hours of cooking and would fill my long days. I cooked southern dishes that I remembered from my childhood and ate double portions of everything. I developed a sweet tooth, consuming things that had never before crossed my lips—packaged doughnuts, cupcakes, and chocolate candy.

It was a vicious cycle. I woke up thinking about food, and I went to sleep thinking about food. I ate all the time. To add to it all, I almost never exercised (except for walks on the beach) which was unusual for me since exercise had always been an integral part of my life. I realized that there was a reason why I had stopped running on the beach and swimming in the ocean—I was embarrassed about how I looked. And, unbelievably, I seemed to have ignored how unattractive my body had become.

It is not my nature to give up, and I decided right then that I wasn't going to do so. I realized that I needed help, and that I needed it quickly. First I called my agent and told him that I couldn't take this part because I needed at least three weeks to get ready. It was one of the hardest things I have ever had to do, but I knew that I had to take care of myself before I could go on with my life. I had to take my life into my own hands, and I was determined to succeed, not only for the next good part that might come along, but for myself.

I got the name of a nutritionist from my doctor and went to see her the next day. It was much more traumatic than I thought it would be. I had not considered what it would be like to talk to someone about what had obviously become a problem; I had not come to terms with the fact that taking off this weight would be hard work and would not be accomplished with the touch of a magic wand.

I casually told the nutritionist that I had gained some weight and needed to talk to her about how best to lose it, but I refused to get on the scale. We talked about how and why my weight had ballooned, and adjourned until the next visit, which was to be a week later.

I returned home and immediately went on a crash diet, knowing full well that the next week I would have to get on the scale—and I didn't want to weigh in at over 140 pounds. My version of a crash diet was to stop eating.

If I only knew then what I know now! But I didn't, so I did what most people do when they are desperate—I simply did not eat. I drank gallons of black coffee. I felt awful—sick, nervous, dizzy, the works.

I woke up in the morning asking God to help me stay on my so-called "diet." During the next week food was always on my mind; it overshadowed everything else. I alternated between feeling elated that I was going to get help and feeling totally defeated at the prospect of having to lose that weight. At times I couldn't imagine looking as good as I had once looked—I believed that that me might be gone forever.

When I went in to see the nutritionist the following week, I weighed in at 139 pounds. But I looked and felt so terrible that this time, finally, I knew I needed her help.

And help me she did. She explained that my overeating had come from my unhappiness with myself, that eating had taken an importance in my life that was out of proportion, that I could and would stop this obsession. She taught me that I had to have a plan, that I needed to find a way of eating that was both comfortable and healthy. She explained that I needed to learn what was in the foods I was eating and how these nutrients or "poisons" affected not only my weight but my health as well. And she assured me that this was possible.

It was. I began a nutritional program that helped me lose weight and taught me a whole new way of living.

I've come a long way since that day at the beach. Today I consider the health of my body to be my most valuable asset, and I don't abuse it. I get enough sleep, I exercise as much as I can, and I eat well. Now I would no more knowingly feed garbage to my body than I would put tar in the gas tank of my car. I *choose* to give my body nourishing food rather than to pollute it. The choice, after all, is mine.

Now, I am not obsessive about eating nutritiously, at least not to the point where I feel controlled by the food I eat or deprived of eating what I like. On the contrary, I feel that *I* am in control of what I eat—and that is a wonderful feeling! I eat a piece of cake when I want to and do so without regret or guilt, but I don't eat two or three pieces at a sitting and I compensate by balancing the cake with a healthier meal the next time around (but more about moderation and balancing later). And, I don't think about what I should and should not eat when I get up in the morning.

Through the knowledge I have gained about what is in what we eat, I am at least aware of and sensible about what I put in my body. Remember, we really are what we eat. The food I digest affects my physical health, my energy, my temperament, and my life. It also directly affects how my body looks, how it works, how it feels, and how long it is going to be around.

In my first book, *The Body Principal,* in the chapter on the relationship between food and a healthy body, I quoted Mark Twain: "Part of the secret of success in life is to eat what you like and let the food fight it out inside." We now know that doesn't work. In fact, today many of us are quite aware of the importance of good nutrition to our general health—it's hard not to be when daily newspaper headlines read "Obesity Kills" or "Additional Bad News about Sodium!"

We have heard that foods with additives are not good for us, that too much salt adversely affects our blood pressure and can often increase water retention, that fats cause increased and unwanted amounts of cholesterol (not to mention weight) in the body. But often all this information about the dangers of some foods, and advice on what to do about all the pro's and con's of nutrition, is confusing and overwhelming.

For nearly every theory on food and the body, there is an expert to agree with or refute it. There is good cholesterol and bad cholesterol. You need some minerals, but an excess of one can drain you of another. Vitamins are necessary, but not if they are used as a substitute for eating well. And how much you need of each vitamin is yet another daily debate.

Margarine vs. butter; processed sugar vs. raw sugar; white flour vs. wheat flour; proteins with carbohydrates vs. proteins without carbohydrates; caffeine in coffee is bad, caffeine in tea is not-so-bad. The Food and Drug Administration (FDA) suggests certain Recommended Daily Dietary Allowances (RDA's) for vitamins and nutrients, but many people (even some doctors) do not agree that these are correct. Besides, when was the last time you weighed your food to check if you were getting a sufficient amount of RDA's? It's enough to make you scream: "Enough!"

But instead of screaming, I have tried over the years to simplify it all for myself. I have discussed diets and nutrition with doctors and nutritionists. I have read about nutrition and diets, and have gained (pardon the expression) a knowledge of what foods do to my body. By paying attention to what I eat (I don't mean being compulsive and writing down every piece of food that crosses my lips!) and by observing the effects of these foods on my own body, I have found which foods keep me healthy, which let me lose weight comfortably and permanently, and which just plain do me wrong.

I have developed a nutritious way of eating—a "diet," if you will—that has enabled me to maintain my weight and to eat sensibly and enjoyably. Now, let's get one thing out of the way—when I say diet, I don't mean just "losing weight." In fact, I often think that "diet" has become one of those unmentionable four-letter words that make the listener cringe and shudder, much like the sound of chalk on the board.

I use the word "diet" to mean *a nutritional way of eating*. In this book there is a diet for life (some people call this a maintenance diet) and there are two diets to lose weight.

The Diet for Life will educate you about eating—it is the sensible (and you could say delicious) way you will eat well for the rest of your life. The 30-Day Diet to Lose is a commonsense way of eating nutritionally and losing weight at the same time. I have also developed the Bikini Diet for those special, emergency times when that extra weight just has to come off quickly, yet safely.

The Diet Principal is all this, and more. It is full of principles that will help you understand how to deal with food and "dieting" in your life. It is full of information that you can "digest" so you will know what is in what you eat. It contains a list of those foods that are forbidden (don't worry, it's a pretty short list) and a list of those that are perfect for you. And it is full of advice on how to eat well easily, enjoyably, and happily. Now don't panic—you don't have to memorize all this information. But I guarantee you that once you read it, you will remember the basics and will be on your way to eating well for the rest of your life.

Much of this information comes from my years of studying and soaking up any and all the data and theories on food and nutrition that have come my way. Some information comes from reports of the Food and Drug Administration, some from the Department of Agriculture, some from nutritionists and medical doctors, and some from my friends who have been trying my "diets" in their various forms for many years.

And thus this book. The purpose of *The Diet Principal* is twofold: it is about nutrition and eating for life, and it is about losing weight sensibly, safely, and easily. It is not a fad-diet book·—the diets are not harmful to your health. Rather, it is a book for the modern woman who wants to take control of her life. It is for you—you know that taking care of yourself is of primary importance, and you need a nutritious program of eating that lets you lose or maintain your weight so that you are always healthy, a program that provides the flexibility your life demands.

I consider myself to be a modern woman with a hectic schedule that demands great organization and a lot of stamina. When I am working on "Dallas" I have to be on the set at six o'clock in the morning. Often I don't get home before seven o'clock at night. That doesn't leave me very much time for the business of running my life. But I do maintain my own household and do all my own cooking. Thus I don't have time for complicated meals or eating habits—weighing foods, measuring for nutritional content, worrying about how much or how little I should be eating (whether it's at home or in a restaurant).

The Diet Principal was written for you. By making the Diet Principles an integral and habitual part of your life, by following the Diet to Lose when you want to lose weight and the Diet for Life for the rest of your life, you will assure that your body will be at its healthiest, fittest, and most beautiful—the best it can be, always.

PRINCIPLE ONE:
Start forming healthy eating habits today!

It is never too late to learn how to eat in a healthy manner. And it is important to learn good eating habits: how to avoid excesses, how to eat in moderation, and how to recognize changes in your life and their possible effects on your eating habits.

PRINCIPLE TWO:
Know what's in what you eat.

You need to educate yourself about the foods you eat. Learn what is in what you eat, what you need for good nutrition, and how to avoid gaining unnecessary and unhealthy weight. Learn how food is digested, how vitamins and minerals affect your body; learn what damage can be caused by an excess of fat, salt, and other potentially harmful substances. When you have even a small amount of basic scientific knowledge about the relationship between food and your body, you can then learn how to eat properly and healthily.

PRINCIPLE THREE:
Understand why you eat too much.

Analyze your eating habits and patterns so you can understand your eating style. Such an understanding of your eating life is the basis for making successful changes. You may need to change your outlook about food and eating, and to learn to have more respect for what you put into your body. Permanent retraining may be in order.

PRINCIPLE FOUR:
Don't hide behind your weight; losing weight has to be a goal in itself—you have to be motivated to lose that weight.

Many people who are overweight hide behind their weight. The extra pounds shield their real feelings, cover their vulnerabilities, and protect them from the outside world. Such people may also use this weight as an excuse for why they cannot succeed in life.

You can avoid this problem by being realistic in your expectations about what losing weight can do for you; then make losing weight your goal. Losing weight *will* make you a healthier person; it *will* most probably make you more attractive to yourself and to others. But it *will not* make you a millionaire; it will not solve all your personal problems; it will not create relationships where none exist.

Losing that weight *will* remove that barrier behind which you have been hiding; it could help you remake your self-image and build up your self-esteem, your own sense of yourself. By taking control of your weight, you may then find that you have the strength to deal with your other personal problems and challenges.

PRINCIPLE FIVE:
Moderation and balance are the key to a successful diet.

I don't believe in total or constant self-denial because such an attitude will not result in any permanent and healthy weight loss. In the short run, denying yourself certain pleasurable foods may work, but to promise that you will never again eat chocolate cake is unrealistic, because chances are great you won't be able to live up to such a promise. And if you can't, then you will eat the cake and feel guilty, and then where are you? Self-denial is useless, and unnecessary. As long as you understand that moderation is the key to dieting successfully, you can almost assuredly eat your favorite dishes at least once in a while.

I am also against self-imposed starvation, because it can be very harmful to your body and because it is a temporary measure that does not work in the long run. Remember, the point is to establish a lifetime of good eating, starting with a sensible and workable reducing diet followed by an eating plan that is forever. The idea is to take the best care of your body that you possibly can now, to routinely put the best fuel into your body so that you will look and feel the best you can.

PRINCIPLE SIX:
Dieting is a positive, not a negative.

Diet for Life means not being a hermit. And "not eating food" shouldn't be the center of your day or of your life. You do not have to withdraw from life while you diet. If you become obsessed with eating, with gaining or losing weight, whatever you do to your body will be both temporary and probably unhealthy. Understand that while the ceremony around food can be fun, eating is not a reward but a simple daily occurrence that is necessary for a healthy body. Food should not take on undue importance in your daily life.

PRINCIPLE SEVEN:
Learn the difference between dieting to lose weight and dieting as a nutritious way of eating to maintain weight.

Understand what "diet" means: there is a diet to lose weight, and there is a diet (manner of eating) to maintain your weight for the rest of your life. Diet is *what you eat*—it is not denial of eating. Dieting should not be a fad, or an obsession. It should be merely an understanding of how to eat well, a dedication to taking care of your body, and a commitment to making healthful eating, whether it is to lose or to maintain your weight, a simple habitual part of your life.

PRINCIPLE EIGHT:
Be flexible!

Remember to be flexible enough to change. You don't have to be adamant about eating or not eating certain foods (except for the absolutely "forbidden foods," and there are only a few of those). You need to know what your body is telling you—when losing weight is a good idea, when it is a bad time to put additional stress on your system, when your body weight is ideal and when it is not. You need to recognize that at different times in your life your body may need different care. For example, at times of stress, at times of menstruation or pregnancy, your body needs different nutrients than at other times. So be flexible about these changes.

PRINCIPLE NINE:
Know thyself—be the best that you can be, not the best that someone else may be.

Never try to look like someone else. Know your own comfortable and healthy body-weight. Don't decide that because your best friend looks great at 105 pounds, this is the ideal weight for you. Your ideal weight depends on a lot of things—on your general health; on your body size, or frame and build; on your weight history; and sometimes on your age. Learn to know your body and realistically recognize at which weight you are most comfortable, at which you feel and look your best. Then you can safely and intelligently diet to meet that weight and to maintain it.

PRINCIPLE TEN:
Make a commitment to yourself.

Take charge of your life. Learn to deal with temptation. Make exercising and eating right a permanent way of life—a new, serious, and permanent commitment.

An added note: I am not a doctor, nor am I a nutritionist. I can only tell you how this program of eating healthy foods in certain combinations and quantities has helped me and many of my friends. But I do believe that before embarking on a *new* program of nutrition—particularly if it is to lose that extra weight—you need professional advice. Just as you would go to a lawyer for advice on a legal problem, so I urge you see a doctor and/or a nutritionist before you embark on any diet. Many people have found the 30-Day Diet to Lose and the Diet for Life to be the perfect balanced and effective eating-program. But individuals are just that—individuals—with different health problems and personal medical characteristics. So make the program really safe for yourself—see a doctor before you begin.

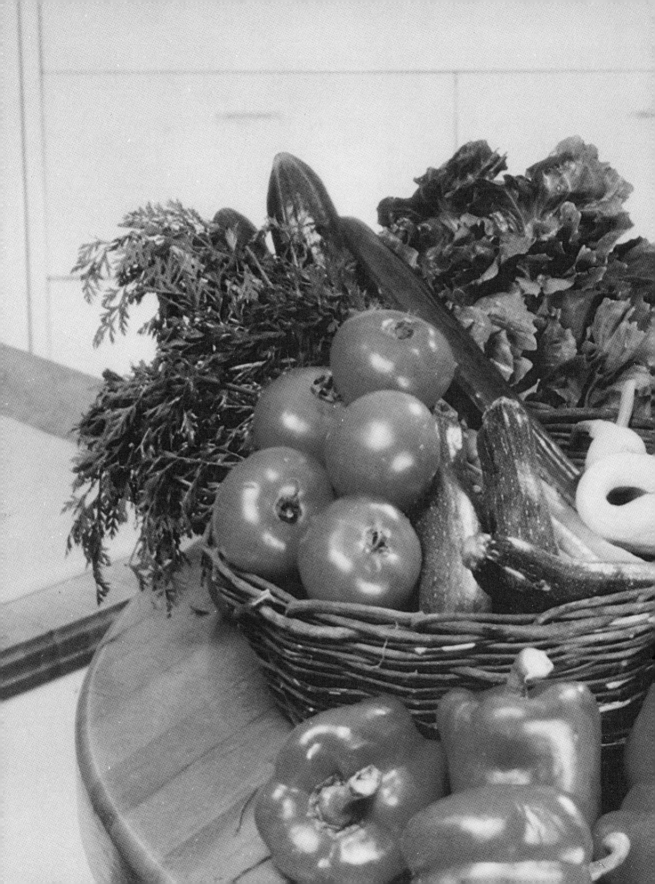

CHAPTER 2

NUTRITION: WHAT'S IN WHAT WE EAT

In the past, the word "diet" conjured up in my mind visions of obsessive behavior; of great longing for untouchable foods; of need, hunger denial, and deprivation; and particularly of a demand to give everything up. Every time I saw the word "diet" anywhere, I saw food.

Now, if you want to healthfully and permanently lose weight or merely to maintain your ideal weight, seeing the word that challenges and taunts you at every turn is truly counterproductive. Thus I have taught myself to redefine diet to mean "a nutritional way of eating," which immediately eliminates its pejorative connotation and takes away some of the pain of hearing it everywhere. So from now on, "diet" means not how little you can eat, but *how* and *what* you eat.

And that is the crux of the matter—what you eat, how much of it you eat, and what's in what you eat determine how much you weigh, how much you lose, and how healthy you are. The most important question you can ask yourself about any food is not "Is this fattening?" but rather "What does this do for my body?"

I truly believe that it is impossible to lose weight, to keep it off, and to stay healthy without having a basic knowledge of nutrition. Once you know what's in what you eat, eating healthy, well-balanced meals both to lose and to maintain your weight will be a piece of . . . apple.

Mae West said, "Too much of a good thing is ecstasy." She was probably right —except for food. Now, I don't believe in extremes of any kind—therefore I don't hold to living a life of total denial. I gave up feeling guilty about eating chocolate cake a long time ago; I don't kick myself for eating an occasional hamburger with everything on it; and I have not yet vowed that a slice of pizza will never again pass my lips.

I do believe, however, that eating any of these things excessively or regularly as part of a *diet for life* can be detrimental to your health. And if your goal is to lose weight, you're going to need to exercise some control over what you eat, until you reach your ideal weight. My theory is, if I leave out the forbidden foods, occasionally eat the questionable foods, and try to concentrate on eating the healthy foods, I'll be ahead of the game by a long shot. Merely eating less is a start but it's not the only answer—it's eating nutritious food in a balanced combination so your body gets all the nutrients it needs. Remember, you can be well fed and not well nourished.

The key, then, is moderation and balance.

Before you can balance the foods in your diet you have to understand how food affects your body, what the body needs to function successfully, and why it is that certain foods are just plain bad for you and should be eliminated from your diet. According to Sandy J. Wickham, who wrote an excellent book called *Human Nutrition: A Self-instructional Text*, nutrition studies have shown "that greater familiarity with different foods and the use of sound principles promote behavioral change and . . . development of beneficial food habits."

Because I am nutritionally aware, every time I look at a slice of salami or bologna I see those little white pieces of fat stacking themselves up in my arteries and making themselves right at home on my thighs. Every time I see a little cellulite on my arms or my legs, it looks like cottage cheese to me. Thus I haven't eaten any of these foods in years, because I know that what is in them should not be in me.

Learning what's in *what* you eat can be complex. My aim here is not to reproduce all available information but to explain as simply as possible why our bodies need nutrients, how these nutrients are utilized by the body, and what is in the foods we so casually devour. Since I have become aware of what is in the foods I eat and how they affect my health, I have been much more careful about what I put into my body. And believe me, such care takes little effort. You'll be surprised at how easy it is to give your body the good fuel it needs rather than the poisons it can do without.

Both the 30-Day Diet to Lose and the Diet for Life have already taken into account all the nutritional ingredients in foods. They are balanced diets, so you don't have to count nutrients, weigh food, or calculate vitamin content every time you prepare a meal. It's all been done for you. The purpose of the food content charts in this chapter is simply to help you learn what is in the foods you eat.

THE THINGS WE NEED

Food is fuel for the body. Without it, the body cannot function or survive. Explains Dr. Paul Ward, Director of Research and Program Development for the Health and Tennis Corporation of America: "The body uses food in two ways: one, as a source of fuel for body heat, metabolism, muscular activity, and work; and two, as a source of nutrients for continual repair and maintenance of all tissues. All foods can be used as fuel for energy, but no one food provides all the nutrients needed by the body." This is where balancing your foods comes in.

As you may remember from your first high school science class, the body needs "the big six": vitamins, minerals, proteins, fats, carbohydrates, and water. (Obviously the basic question is, how much of each of these does the body need? But more on that later.) When these are digested, they interact with the enzymes and acids in our bodies to produce, among other things, energy.

Vitamins

The vitamins in our system regulate the metabolic process, helping to build up our tissues and bones and to process the fats, carbohydrates, proteins, and minerals that our bodies need. Vitamins are found in foods and can also be taken in pills as a dietary supplement (but not as a substitute for food).

The charts on pages 29–31 show the government's Recommended Daily Dietary Allowances (RDA's) of vitamins, and the vitamin contents of various foods. Refer to them as you prepare your meals or read articles about the latest nutritional findings. I have found that even my cursory knowledge of food contents stays in my head and crops up conveniently just as I am preparing a meal. Believe me, such information is not burdensome or intrusive—you need it to learn about what you are putting into your body and what your body needs.

The information in the charts is not for you to memorize. When you put it together with information obtained from the Contents of Foods chart, you will be able to judge if you are balancing your meals. For example, you know by reading this chart that you need at least 800 units of vitamin A each day. If you look up broccoli in the Contents of Food chart (see p. 11),

VITAMIN RDA'S FOR WOMEN

Ages	VITAMINS								
	A units	D ugs	E mgs	C mgs	B_1 mgs	B_2 mgs	B_3 mgs	B_{12} mcgs	K mcgs
15–18	800	10	8	60	1.1	1.3	14	3	50–100
19–22	800	7.5	8	60	1.1	1.3	14	3	70–140
23–50	800	5	8	60	1.0	1.2	13	3	70–140
51 +	800	5	8	60	1.0	1.2	13	3	70–140
Pregnant	1000	+5	+2	80	+ .4	+ .3	+ 2	4	70–140

Recommended Daily Dietary Allowances, 1980; Food and Nutrition Board, National Academy of Sciences National Research Council.

FOOD SOURCES OF VITAMINS

VITAMIN	SOURCE	NEEDED FOR
A	fish-liver oils liver and kidneys **green and yellow vegetables** **yellow-fleshed fruits** (peaches, apricots, cantaloupe, papayas, tangerines) **tomatoes** butter and **margarine** egg yolks **carrots**	growth healthy eyes structure and function of cells of skin
B_1 (Thiamine)	**seafood** meat **soybeans** **nonfat milk** **whole grain products** **fowl** pork **pasta** **oatmeal** **lima beans** oysters	growth carbohydrate metabolism functioning of heart, nerves, and muscles

continued

FOOD SOURCES OF VITAMINS

VITAMIN	SOURCE	NEEDED FOR
B$_2$ (Riboflavin)	meat **soybeans** milk **(nonfat)** **green vegetables** eggs **fowl** **yeast** **whole grain products** **pasta** **mushrooms** **dried beans and peas**	growth healthy skin carbohydrate metabolism functioning of pancreas sugar control functioning of eyes

B$_3$ (Niacin)	meat
	fowl
	fish
	peanut butter (low oil)
	potatoes
	tomatoes
	leafy vegetables
	tuna
	eggs
	whole grain products
	dried peas and beans
		carbohydrate metabolism
		stomach, intestinal, and
		   nervous system
		   functioning

B$_{12}$	**green vegetables** liver meat eggs **fish** milk **(nonfat)** kidneys	preventing anemia feeling sensations
C	**citrus and other fruits** **tomatoes** **leafy vegetables** **potatoes**	strength of blood vessels teeth and gum development growth

VITAMIN	SOURCE	NEEDED FOR
D	liver fortified milk **(nonfat)** eggs	growth calcium and phosphorus metabolism bone and tooth maintenance
E	**wheat germ** butter and **margarine** **green leafy vegetables** **whole grain products** **bread** **dried beans** liver	normal reproduction energy
K	**green vegetables** **tomatoes** soybean oil **cabbage** **cauliflower** **potatoes** **cereals**	normal clotting of blood normal liver functions

*Note: Those foods printed in **bold** are the foods preferred for use as a vitamin source. For example, for a source of vitamin A you would do better to use the yellow and green vegetables instead of butter or egg yolks, which contain fat that you don't need or want.*

you'll find that one cup of cooked broccoli has about 3800 units of vitamin A. Thus you will always know that eating one cup of broccoli gives you more than enough of your daily requirement of vitamin A.

Minerals

Minerals are also found in the foods we eat (particularly in vegetables and meats) and act to regulate the chemical reactions in our cells. They are crucial for adequate muscle contractions and form part of the enzyme system that ensures proper functioning of the body. Explains noted nutritionist Hermien Lee: "Minerals needed by the body can be classified in two types: one group are the macrominerals which you need in large amounts (these include calcium, potassium, phosphorus, magnesium, sodium, sulfur, and chloride). The microminerals are those we need in minute amounts and get easily in our foods (and thus we are not as concerned with accounting for these when we plan diets). These include iron, zinc, manganese, copper, iodine, and others."

A balanced diet will generally give us all the minerals we need (except for iron and calcium, minerals many women need to plan for).

FOOD SOURCES OF MINERALS

MINERAL	SOURCE	NEEDED FOR
Calcium	**Parmesan cheese**	bones and teeth
	nonfat or low-fat dairy products	muscle contraction
	cream	blood clotting
	whole milk	cell membranes
	cheese	
	green leafy vegetables	
	bone meal	
	sardines	
	canned salmon (with bones)	
	citrus fruits	
	dried beans	
Phosphorus	**Parmesan cheese**	bones and teeth
	nonfat or low-fat dairy products	formation of cell membranes and enzymes
	fish	
	poultry	
	meat	

MINERAL	SOURCE	NEEDED FOR
Phosphorus (cont.)	cream whole milk cheese eggs **nuts** **bone meal** **dried beans**	
Magnesium	**nuts** **whole grains** **green leafy vegetables** **fish**	bones making proteins nervous system
Iron	meat eggs **green leafy vegetables** **whole grains** **dried fruit** **dried beans**	supply oxygen to cells proteins and enzymes
Zinc	meat **fish** eggs **chicken**	makes up enzymes
Iodine	iodized salt **fish**	functioning of thyroid reproduction

Potassium	**dried fruits**
	orange juice
	bananas
	meat
	peanut butter (no oil)
	dried beans
	potatoes
	vegetables
		muscle contraction
		release of energy from
		    proteins, fats, and
		    carbohydrates
		nervous system

MINERAL RDA'S FOR WOMEN

	MINERALS							
Age	Cal mg	Phos mg	Mag mg	Iron mg	Zinc mg	Iod mg	Potass mg	Sod mg
15–18	1200	1200	300	18	15	150	1900–5800	3300**
19–22	800*	800	300	18	15	150	1900–5800	3300**
23–50	800*	800	300	18	15	150	1900–5800	3300**
51 +	800*	800	300	10	15	150	1900–5800	3300**
Pregnant	+ 400	+ 400	+ 150	supp	+ 5	+ 25	1900–5800	3300**

* These figures are from 1980. Recent study results have pointed out the importance of a higher calcium intake in preventing osteoporosis. Most doctors now believe that all women should consume at least 1200 mgs of calcium each day.

** The recommended intake for sodium is 3300 mgs, but most physicians will tell you that an intake of about 1100–2300 mgs is more than enough.

Recommended Daily Dietary Allowances, 1980; Food and Nutrition Board, National Academy of Sciences National Research Council.

The following charts indicate how much our bodies need of each mineral and which foods contain these minerals. The charts include those minerals we need to be concerned about and omit trace minerals we get routinely. Two of the minerals most important to women, calcium and iron, will be discussed separately, as will the big one we really don't love or want much of—sodium (see p. 53).

A Word about Calcium

Chances are you've heard or read a lot about calcium lately— how women need extra calcium to combat osteoporosis (a bone disease that often occurs in women over the age of forty), how our diets don't always provide enough calcium, and how important calcium supplements are in our daily diets. I believe wholeheartedly that this is all true and that the importance of calcium cannot be emphasized enough. Although statistics vary, doctors believe that at least 9 million women in this country suffer from osteoporosis, and many more women will get the disease since they are already suffering from a cumulative deficiency of calcium.

Calcium is the structural matter found in bones and teeth. It also helps blood clotting, thereby preventing hemorrhaging. It contracts muscles, helps move impulses along the nerves, and even helps the heart beat properly. Calcium also plays a part in the give and take in the enzyme and hormonal systems in our bodies.

Hermien Lee explains, "Our bodies store calcium in the bones in the spine until we are in our mid-twenties, and in the arms and legs until the mid-thirties. During this time, whenever the body needs calcium for other functions, it acts much like a reliable customer at a bank—it withdraws as much calcium as it needs."

The potential problems in this system are obvious. As long as you get enough calcium in your diet, chances are that the calcium reserve in your bones will be sufficient to handle all those withdrawals. But what's enough calcium? The National Institutes of Health recently recommended that the calcium RDA for women be increased. Up until menopause women need 1000–1500 milligrams of calcium a day, except during pregnancy when they supply calcium to their growing fetuses and need at least 1200 mgs. a day; after menopause women need 1400 mgs. a day. But, says Dr. Sandra Aronberg, most women normally get only about 500 mgs. a day from their diet (primarily because most calcium is found in dairy products, and many women have quit drinking all that milk and stopped eating that fat-laden food known as cheese); that means they don't have enough calcium in reserve. Here's where the trouble starts. When the calcium account in your bones is overdrawn, the bones become thinner and weaker, and can easily break.

There is also good news, however. According to Dr. Aron-

CALCIUM-RICH FOODS

FOOD	QUANTITY	CALCIUM (MGS)
Milk, low-fat, nonfat	1 cup	300
Cottage cheese	½ cup	77
Yogurt (low-fat or nonfat)	1 cup	415
Ice cream, vanilla	1 cup	176
Sardines (with bones)	⅓ cup	372
Canned salmon (with bones)	⅓ cup	167
Broccoli	1 stalk	158
Spinach, cooked	1 cup	200
Almonds	½ cup	166
Tortilla (wheat- or corn-flour)	2	120
Molasses	1 Tablespoon	137
Orange (sections)	1 cup	74

berg, there are studies that suggest large doses of calcium may actually halt the terrible effects of calcium deficiency. Merely taking a calcium supplement of 1000 mgs. a day in the form of a pill easily ensures that you get your daily dose of this much needed mineral. (You can occasionally take two Tums, which each have 500 mgs. of calcium and don't contain any sodium.

Other Calcium Tips

1. Exercise—explains Dr. Paul Ward: "Exercise puts stress on your bones, which means they become stronger and are less susceptible to breakage."

2. Give up coffee—besides the bad effects of caffeine (see section "Things We Don't Need," page 45), it also drains the body of calcium. If you must have it, add low-fat or nonfat milk.

3. For extra calcium, use yogurt in salad dressing, and Parmesan cheese instead of margarine on vegetables (2 tablespoons of grated Parmesan cheese add 69 mgs. of calcium to your diet—plus it's the one cheese I allow on the Diet for Life because it has almost no fat).

4. Make salmon salad a substitute for tuna as often as possible—it's a wonderful food, laden with calcium and potassium.

5. Stay away from *sodium*—more on this later, but be aware that in addition to its other bad characteristics sodium is excreted from the body with calcium. Thus the more sodium you excrete, the more calcium you lose.

6. Lest we get too complicated here, just know that there is a relationship between phosphorus and calcium—too much phosphorus can contribute to loss of calcium. All you have to do is avoid those foods I urge you to forget about anyway—red meat, colas, and processed foods.

7. Sorry, but it's true—alcohol diminishes calcium absorption into the body. This doesn't mean you have to avoid alcohol altogether on the Diet for Life (you do forget about its existence on the 30-Day Diet to Lose, for caloric reasons), but it does mean that you should never take a calcium pill with alcohol (that may sound funny, but just think of the times you may be at a restaurant and decide to take your supplement while you drink your dinner wine!).

8. Some studies suggest that there is evidence that a diet high in calcium and in potassium can lower high blood-pressure. Whether or not this is an accurate finding, potassium is still a very important mineral. Thus the following list of foods that contain both calcium and potassium:

POTASSIUM AND CALCIUM

FOOD	QUANTITY	POTASSIUM (MG)	CALCIUM (MG)
Banana	1	550	12
Broccoli	1 stalk	414	136
Brussels sprouts	1 cup	423	50
Cantaloupe	½ cup	682	38
Chicken breast	1 lb	1630	39
Chicken thigh	1 lb	1630	41
Grapefruit juice	1 cup	405	22
Halibut	1 lb	2037	59
Honeydew melon	1 cup	377	21
Lima beans, cooked	1 cup	1163	55
Milk, low-fat/nonfat	1 cup	406	302
Orange juice	1 cup	496	27
Parsley, fresh	1 cup	436	122
Peas, cooked split	1 cup	592	22
Potato, baked	1	782	32
Salmon, canned	1 cup	794	431
Soybeans, cooked	½ cup	972	131
Spinach, cooked	1 cup	583	167
Sweet potato, canned	1 cup	400	50
Turkey, white meat	1 lb	1864	36
Veal cutlet	1 lb	1157	41
Yogurt, nonfat plain	1 cup	531	415

A Word about Iron

Mother said there'd be days like this—remember? Every month during menstruation many women feel tired and sluggish, a feeling partially due to loss of iron. Generally, a woman doesn't need iron supplements unless she is pregnant or anemic (as diagnosed by a doctor, not by herself). But it is helpful and important at all times to eat foods rich in iron, especially because most women who limit their daily calorie intake in any way may also be denying themselves the iron they need.

Explains Dr. Aronberg, "The typical diet of the American woman results in a consumption of about 1500 calories a day.

Since we typically calculate that a normal diet provides about 6 mgs. of iron for every 1000 calories, a woman on the 1500-calorie-a-day program will be getting only half of the recommended 18 mgs. of iron a day."

Thus it is important to try to eat foods high in iron every day. Again, let me repeat that a balanced diet composed of the foods recommended for the Diet for Life will contain a sufficient daily intake of iron. The following chart of foods high in iron is presented merely for your information, not for you to memorize.

IRON-RICH FOODS*

FOOD	MGS PER 3-OUNCE SERVING
Almonds	4.7
Apple (one small)	.3
Apricots, dried	5.5
Bananas	.7
Beef, hamburger	3.5
Bread, whole wheat, 1 slice	.5
Chicken, dark meat	2.0
Cod, broiled	1.0
Eggs, poached	2.2
Lima beans, cooked	2.5
Liver, cooked	8.8
Oysters, canned	8.1
Peas	2.5
Prune juice	4.1
Raisins	3.5
Soybeans, cooked	2.5
Spinach	2.0
Tuna	1.9
Wheat cereal	4.4

Note: Foods in **bold** are recommended on the Diet for Life.
* Chart excerpted from Sandy J. Wickham, Human Nutrition: A Self-instructional Text (Bowie, Maryland: Robert J. Brady Company, 1982).

Protein

Protein is everywhere in our bodies. Dr. Ward states, "Every cell in the body is made up of some protein. Protein is part of you in every way—it is in your muscles, bones, blood, skin, and lymph system. As a matter of fact, all the enzymes in your body are protein—so it's not as if your body is starving for it."

But we cannot exist without protein. Explains Dr. Ward, "To put it as simply as possible, protein is essential for the body's ability to form new tissues and repair ones that are worn out. It is necessary to make the antibodies without which we could not fight diseases, and is crucial to the body's ability to clot blood and to form scar tissue. (As a matter of fact, protein contains amino acids which are the basic building blocks for tissue maintenance, growth, and repair.) Protein is the carrier of nutrients and oxygen in the blood, and makes up the cell membranes and the nucleus."

You may be surprised to learn that we Americans routinely eat a lot more protein than we need. Explains Hermien Lee, "The American diet is chock full of protein, most of which we don't need. Excess protein in the body means extra calories which in turn means all you get is extra weight. This is particularly true in our diets, which are high in fat (because much of our complete protein comes from animal meat) and in calories."

Although it is the "complete" proteins from animal meat which provide those essential amino acids in the right proportion for use in the body, so-called "incomplete" proteins from vegetables can be combined in a way to effectively nourish the body. What is important about complete protein is that you don't have to get it from meat high in fat—you can combine the incomplete proteins found in vegetables to form a complete protein.

This is much simpler than it sounds. All it means is that

PROTEIN IN COMMON FOODS

FOOD	PORTION	PROTEIN (GMS)
Beans		
Kidney	½ cup	7.2
Lima	½ cup	6.5
Navy	½ cup	7.4
Bologna	3 slices	10.2
American cheese	1 slice	6.6
Cottage cheese	½ cup	15.0
Chicken	1 drumstick	12.2
Eggs	2	11.4
Fish		
Canned salmon	3 ounces	17.0
Scallops	6	16.0
Tuna (water)	1 cup	56
Trout	½ pound	48.5
Bass	½ pound	43.0
Halibut	½ pound	47.0
Hot Dog	1	7.0
Ham	3 ounces	18.0
Hamburger meat	¼ pound	23.4
Lentils	½ cup	7.8
Macaroni (pasta)	1 cup cooked	6.5
Milk (low/nonfat)	1 cup	8.0
Peanut butter (low oil)	2 tablespoons	8.0
Peas, Green	½ cup cooked	4.3
Pizza, Cheese	2 slices	15.6
Pork	3 ounces	20.8
Potato	1 baked	4.0
Rice, brown	1 cup cooked	4.9
Spaghetti	1 cup cooked	6.5
Yogurt, low fat plain	1 cup	12.0

Data from "Nutritive Value of American Foods in Common Units," by Catherine F. Adams, U.S. Department of Agriculture Handbook No. 456, Nov. 1975.

instead of eating a steak once a day (which will give you the protein you need but will also clog your arteries with its high fat content), you can combine vegetables and beans, or beans and rice, to easily get enough protein.

Now in case you've decided that you have to wake up every morning and plan for your protein intake of the day—forget it! Chances are you'll be getting all the protein you need from the fish, milk products, eggs, and chicken you eat regularly. Just be aware that certain foods are both high in protein and low in fat, and therefore better for you.

To calculate how much protein you need every day, multiply your weight in pounds by .36 grams (if you are pregnant, multiply by .62 grams). For example, I weigh 110 pounds and need 39.6 grams of protein daily.

The chart on page 41 is presented to familiarize you with good sources of protein. All the foods listed contain more than 4 grams of protein per serving.

Fats

Then there are the fats (talk about four-letter words!). Contrary to what many of us think, fats are essential to our health —it's how much fat we need that is the question. Besides insulating our bodies from the weather, fats serve as a source of energy and carry certain vitamins throughout our system. But the amount of the fat that our bodies need—called poly-unsaturated fat—is minimal and routinely available in nearly everything we eat. It is the saturated fats that we eat too much of, especially since the body does not need these *at all!*

Here are some simple clues to the mystery of fat. Explains Hermien Lee; "We are all born with a number of fat cells, and when we are young, if we eat a lot, we accumulate a lot of fat. (This doesn't mean that all fat babies will be fat adults— although it does bode well for thin babies who almost always turn out to be svelte grown-ups!). Throughout our lives, as we eat, fat is absorbed and stored in these cells. This is fine because some fat is necessary for good health. The trouble begins when the body gets *too much fat.*" The rest of the story on fat contains no good news, so I am saving it for the section "Things We Don't Need" (see pg. 45).

Carbohydrates

Carbohydrates are essential to our health since they are our main source of fuel. We get carbohydrates from cereals, fruits, vegetables, pasta, and breads. Our central nervous system operates almost exclusively on carbohydrates—an inadequate supply would limit endurance in exercise and would also hamper the functioning of our nervous system and brain.

Before you get carried away with the importance of noodles in your life, hang on a minute—you should know that there is more than one kind of carbohydrate. Explains Dr. Ward, "Nutritionists often divide carbohydrates into two groups—*natural* or *'complex'* carbohydrates (the 'good' guys) which are starches, and *processed* or *'refined'* carbohydrates (the very 'bad' guys), which are sugars. The complex carbohydrates (found in fruits and vegetables and whole grain products) are more desirable because they convert into blood sugar slowly, and supply us with vitamins, minerals, and roughage. The bad guys—those sugars and colas and white breads and sugary cereals—are essentially empty calories and low in nutritional value. Because they are rapidly converted into glucose, they cause blood sugar imbalances and are responsible for lots of different ailments (from tooth decay to diabetes to heart disease)." (For further information on sugar, see page 50.)

Heard enough? Just one more thing. Fiber, that roughage that is essential for proper elimination of wastes, is a carbohydrate—a good one. Fiber is found in beans, whole grains, fruits, and vegetables.

Since we do need some complex carbohydrates, how much is "some" and where should we get it from? According to the U.S. Department of Agriculture, women between the ages of 22 and 45, weighing between 110 and 143 pounds, need 270–330 grams of carbohydrates daily. The foods in the following chart are good carbohydrate sources, and they are all recommended on the Diet for Life.

FOOD SOURCES OF CARBOHYDRATES

FOOD	AMOUNT	CARBOHYDRATES (GRAMS)
Apple, raw	1	24
Apple juice (no sugar)	1 cup	29.5
Applesauce (no sugar)	1 cup	26.4
Apricots, dried	1 cup	86.5
Banana	1	33.3
Bran flakes	1 cup	28.2
Cream of Wheat cereal	1 cup	28.2
Dates, pitted	10	72.9
Figs, dried	5	69.1
Graham cracker	1	10.4
Granola	1 cup	57
Lentils, cooked	1 cup	38.6
Lima beans, cooked	1 cup	48.6
Macaroni, cooked	1 cup	32.2
Muffin, whole wheat	1	20.9
Nectarine	1	23.6
Noodles, cooked	1 cup	37.3
Orange	1	16
Orange juice (no sugar)	1 cup	25.8
Peach, dried	1 cup	109
Pear, dried	1 cup	121
Peas, split, cooked	1 cup	41.6
Pineapple, fresh	1 cup	21.2
Pineapple juice (no sugar)	1 cup	33.8
Pita bread, whole wheat	1	24
Popcorn, plain	1 cup	10.7
Potatoes, baked in skin	1	32.8
Prunes, dried	1 cup	108
Raisins, packed	1 cup	128
Red kidney beans, cooked	1 cup	39.6
Rice, brown, cooked	1 cup	38.2
Rice, white, cooked	1 cup	49.6
Squash, winter, baked	1 cup	31.6
Sweet potato, baked	1	37
Watermelon	1 slice	38.4
Wheat germ, toasted	1 cup	48
Yams, cooked in skin	1 cup	48.2

Data from "Nutritive Value of American Foods in Common Units," by Catherine F. Adams, U.S. Department of Agriculture Handbook No. 456, Nov. 1975.

Fiber

More and more studies have shown that fiber is necessary for good health. Fiber, or roughage, ensures that the waste in your body (including such harmful substances as fat) will move rapidly out of the body, thereby helping to prevent absorption of some harmful substances, including carcinogens. There are five kinds of fiber, and all are available in those foods I have listed as being good for you in every way (see page 77). These foods include cereals, vegetables, and fruits. You can also add to your fiber intake by sprinkling coarsely ground bran on any and all foods. It really can't hurt you (in moderation, of course), and the benefits of a cleaner system are undeniable.

Water

Finally there is water, without which the body cannot survive. Water is needed for nearly all our body processes (60% of our body weight is water) and is especially important for temperature regulation. Water, explains Ms. Wickham, "is the medium in which body chemical reactions occur and is the transporter of necessary materials to the cells and metabolic wastes from the cells." Water is found in meats, fruits, and vegetables. But the body needs more water than you can find in these foods, so yes, you do need to drink at least 8 glasses of water (or my own favorite, iced tea) a day.

THE THINGS WE DON'T NEED

Someone once said to me, "You *can* have everything." But the lesson we all have to learn some time is that we may not *need* it all. As a matter of fact, there are times when less *is* more. I don't need extra fat—it will only clog my arteries, pad and inflate my body, and otherwise endanger my health. I don't need that sugar or sodium, those nitrates and nitrites, or an overdose of caffeine. And I learned a long time ago that just a little alcohol will go a long way.

I don't believe in a life of total denial. But there is a smart way to live, and that doesn't include deliberately putting things into your body that you know will only harm you both in the short and long run. And, anyway, when you think about it, these unnecessary and potentially harmful parts of our diets are not worth the price we pay. Once you know how damaging cholesterol, sodium, sugar, and an overindulgence in caffeine can be, I guarantee you it will be a lot easier, if not to give them up, at least to minimize and control your intake of these "things you really don't need."

Fat and Cholesterol

A certain amount of fat is necessary for the body to function properly. But diets high in fat are universally considered to be unhealthy. Remember how the body works—as you eat more and more fat, the fat cells "gain weight," and so do you. The more fat you eat, the more fat they store, etc., etc., etc. It is truly a vicious cycle, but one which you can interrupt and redirect.

Fat makes you fat. Sounds simplistic, but it's very true. Ounce for ounce, fat has twice as many calories as protein and carbohydrates have. Thus fat is fattening! Both The Diet to Lose and The Diet for Life programs are low in fat. The recipes I have been using over the years do not contain too much fat and take into account the fats that exist naturally in foods. Here are some examples of how to reduce fat in your diet:

- Try not to eat red meat; it is unbelievably high in fat. If you like, you can eat veal once in a while because it has less fat than other red meats.

- Always take the skin off chicken. A whole frying chicken usually has about 2000 calories. If you remove the skin, you're left with about 900 calories. That's quite a difference!

- Remember that the saturated fats are the ones you don't need; the polyunsaturates are fine. Watch your intake of butter and oils—and when you do use margarine or oil, use the polyunsaturated kind.

- Salad dressings are high in fat. Try to use only diet dressings or the ones I list in the Diet to Lose. Always try to use the salad fork trick: Have the dressing on the side, and dip the fork into the dressing before taking a bite of the salad.

- Read the Fat Contents of Food chart, and remember the foods that are really high in fat and the substitutions you can make. For example, the difference between the amount of fat in whole milk and that in nonfat milk is crucial to your health!

Besides being fattening, fat is also dangerous to your health. Few experts will argue that too much fat in the diet is a primary cause of some types of cancer, heart attacks, strokes, and a variety of other diseases. While there is a continuing debate about the dangers of high levels of cholesterol in the blood, the argument generally concerns what level is *too high* and does not question the accepted fact that an elevated cholesterol level is not beneficial for anyone.

Although the cholesterol arguments are sure to rage on for some time, there is a consensus that reducing your fat and

FATS AND CHOLESTEROL*

FOOD	AMOUNT	FAT (GRAMS)	CHOLESTEROL (MGS)	
Bacon, sliced	½ pound	157	499	
Beef				
Ground	1 pound	96.2	307	
Liver	1 pound	17.3	1360	
Porterhouse steak	1 pound	148	261	
Bran flakes	1 cup	.6	0	
Brownie	1	9.4	25.5	
Butter	1 tablespoon	11.5	35	
Cake, sponge	1 slice	2.9	123	
Cheese				
American, processed	1 ounce	8.9	27	
Cheddar, American	1 cup	37.4	119	
Cottage, creamed	1 cup	9.5	31	
Cottage, 2% fat	1 cup	4.4	19†	
Mozzarella	1 ounce	6.1	22	
Parmesan, grated	1 tablespoon	1.5	4	
Cheese soufflé	1 cup	16.2	159	
Chicken				
Breast	½ pound	9	119	
Drumstick	½ pound	15.4	119	
Cornbread	2-inch square	3.2	30	
Crackers, soda	1	.4	0	
Cream				
Half-and-half	1 tablespoon	1.7	6	
Whipping	1 cup	88.1	326	
Custard, baked	1 cup	14.6	278	
Egg				
Fried	1	6.4	312	
Scrambled	1	7.1	314	
White, hard-boiled	1	0	0‡	
English muffin	1	0	0	
Fish				
Crab, steamed	½ pound	4.3	226	
Halibut	½ pound	2.5	114	
Herring	½ pound	14	193	
Lobster	1 pound	8.6	900	ouch!
Salmon, canned pink	1 cup	13	77	
Scallops	½ pound	.5	79	
Shrimp, fresh	½ pound	1.8	340§	

FOOD	AMOUNT	FAT (GRAMS)	CHOLESTEROL (MGS)
Tuna, in water	1 cup	1.6	126
Ham	½ pound	69	159
Hot dog	¼ pound	32.7	77
Ice cream, vanilla	1 cup	14.3	59
Macaroni, cooked	1 cup	1	0
Margarine	1 tablespoon	11.5	0
Mayonnaise	1 tablespoon	11.2	10
Milk			
low-fat	1 cup	4.7	18‖
nonfat	1 cup	.5	4
whole	1 cup	8.2	33
Oil			
Olive	1 tablespoon	14	trace
Peanut	1 tablespoon	14	trace
Sunflower	1 tablespoon	14	trace
Pie			
Apple	1 piece	17.8	156
Meringue	1 piece	14.3	130
Popcorn, plain	1 cup	.7	0
Pudding			
Bread, raisins	1 cup	16.2	170
Rice, raisins	1 cup	8.2	29
Sour cream	1 cup	48.7	102
Turkey, white meat	½ pound	8.8	174
Veal cutlet	½ pound	20	127
Whole wheat bread	1	.7	0
Yogurt			
whole milk, plain	1 cup	7.4	29
low-fat, plain	1 cup	3.5	14
nonfat, plain	1 cup	.4	4

* Data compiled from chart appearing in John D. Kirschmann, Nutritional Almanac Cookbook *(New York: McGraw Hill, 1983).*

† *Want to know why this is not in bold? One cup of this low-fat cottage cheese has 918 mgs. of sodium! As a matter of fact, most low-fat cheeses have a lot of sodium, which is why I don't recommend eating any cheese (except grated Parmesan).*

‡ *The white of the egg also has 3.6 grams protein.*

§ *On the face of it, it looks like I made a mistake with shrimp—look at that cholesterol! But you don't usually eat ½ pound of shrimp at a sitting—it's more like ¼ of a pound, so the cholesterol level goes way down. Besides, ¼ pound of shrimp has only 100 calories, and lots of potassium and calcium. So, on balance, the trade-off is worth it. See, I told you you wouldn't have to give up everything! Now, lobster is a different story.*

‖ *See the difference between low-fat and nonfat milk? It is really worth it to stick to the nonfat.*

cholesterol intake on a daily basis—to less than 300 milligrams a day—is beneficial. This is easier than you think—as a matter of fact, the 30-Day Diet to Lose has little or no unnecessary fat in it, and the Diet for Life has been designed to be low-fat and low-cholesterol.

The chart on pages 48–49 contains a list of foods and their fat and cholesterol contents. Read it carefully—you may find a lot of surprises, like the fact that low-fat plain yogurt has half the fat (and therefore half the cholesterol) of whole milk plain yogurt. Now look at the cheese—see how little cholesterol Parmesan has as compared to the other cheeses? Keep looking! Again, the "better for you" foods are in boldface type.

Sugar

Love sugar? Well, sweet may soon turn sour when you find out that the harm sugar can do to your body far outweighs its momentary highs. Sugar is an additive, a dangerously addictive one. You crave it, you eat it, you get a high burst of energy, then a withdrawal low. Then you crave it some more, you eat it again, and the cycle repeats itself.

Some so-called "natural sugar," like that found in fruit, is not harmful to the body, although some nutritionists believe that three glasses of orange juice a day is too much sugar for most people. But, explains Hermien Lee, refined sugar, the addictive sugar, is nothing but empty calories: It makes you fat (because you eat more calories than your body can burn off), destroys your teeth, can cause serious diseases like diabetes and hypoglycemia, disrupts your metabolism, and makes an addict out of you. The irony is you don't need sugar in your diet—the body converts starches into sugar which is then used for energy.

By now you've gotten the point—refined sugar has no redeeming qualities. But, if it is an addictive "drug," how do you stop eating it? That's a difficult, but not impossible, task —difficult because sugar is found in virtually every food we eat. Walk down the aisle in your grocery store, and look at the cans and cartons—*any* cans and cartons, because chances are they all contain sugar. Fructose, dextrose, corn syrup, honey, or just plain sugar—it's all the same. And sometimes it's hidden—every time you put ketchup on your food, you're eating a teaspoon of sugar. Each time you eat a bowl of cereal (including the so-called "natural" granolas), you are eating too much sugar—60 out of the top 75 cereals sold are from 10–56% sugar. (In *The Body Principal* I recommended eating Cheerios. I have been eating Cheerios for years, mostly because it is only 3% sugar.)

My solution to the sugar dilemma is twofold and simple, and follows my Diet Principal philosophy—moderation. First, I try to cut down on the sugar I can control. For example, I never add sugar to anything—not to a drink, not to anything I am cooking, nor to anything I am eating. By doing that I am immediately and simply leaving out of my diet a lot of sugar I don't need. I never have candy in the house and have developed the wonderful habit of eating fruits (both fresh and dried) as snacks.

Second, I try not to eat foods high in sugar, which means eliminating such foods from my regular diet and not worrying about those foods which may have sugar hidden in them. Occasionally, when I want to have a rich dessert and I'm not on the 30-Day Diet to Lose, I do so without guilt or remorse. But then I compensate and eat a low-calorie meal the next time around.

Basically, I have gotten out of the habit of feeling the need for a sweet taste, although I do use artificial sweetener in my iced tea. A word about artificial sweeteners: I like them; I use them; and I have not been convinced that in the amounts I use, they are harmful to my health. Hermien Lee agrees: "One rat would have to drink 829 diet drinks with saccharin every day of his life to affect any cellular change (like cancer) in his body."

Minimizing sugar in your diet is not that difficult. Try it and

SUGAR IN COMMON FOODS*

FOOD	AMOUNT	SUGAR (TEASPOONS)
Apple pie	1 slice	12
Apricots, dried	4	3
Beer	8 ounces	2
Brown sugar	1 tablespoon	3
Chocolate chip cookie	1	1½
Chocolate milk	8 ounces	5–6
Cola drink	8 ounces	4
Corn flakes	1 cup	4
Dates	5	7
Gum	1 piece	1½
Fudge	1 square	4
Hamburger bun	1	3
Honey	1 tablespoon	3½
Hot fudge sundae	1 dish	16
Ice cream	1 cup	6
Jam	1 tablespoon	3
Jelly doughnut	1	6
Lemon meringue pie	1 slice	10
Maple syrup	1 tablespoon	2
Orange juice	1 cup	5
Peanut brittle	1 piece	3½
Prune juice	½ cup	4
Raisins	1 tablespoon	1½
Sherbet	1 cup	12

* *Chart data compiled from the following: J.A.T. Pennington and H.N. Church,* Bowe's and Church's Food Values of Portions Commonly Used *(Philadelphia: J.B. Lippincott Company, 1980); Sandy J. Wickham,* Human Nutrition: A Self-instructional Text *(Bowie, Maryland: Robert J. Brady Company, 1982); Catherine F. Adams,* Nutritive Value of American Foods in Common Units, *U.S. Dept. of Agriculture Handbook No. 456 (Issued Nov. 1975).*

see. If, however, you find that you are experiencing true withdrawal symptoms, you may have a serious sugar addiction and need to see your doctor immediately.

Sodium

Forty percent of table salt is sodium. It's not that sodium is so terrible—as a matter of fact, sodium is a necessary nutrient. But too much sodium can be lethal, and most of us consume way too much. The RDA for sodium is 1100–3300 milligrams per day (that's about ½ to 1½ teaspoons of salt), and some nutritionists and doctors (and I) prefer a diet consisting of no more than 2000 mgs. of sodium a day. But on the average we consume more than 4000 milligrams a day, and that has led nearly all doctors and nutritionists to scream, "Enough! You are killing yourselves!"

They are right. Excess sodium has been named the culprit in high blood pressure (which affects an estimated 60 million Americans), strokes, and kidney diseases, among others. Women who suffer from premenstrual syndrome (PMS) are often great consumers of sodium (according to Dr. Aronberg, the body retains salt before menstruation, causing irritability, headaches, and the bloating that is so familiar to PMS sufferers).

So who needs that much sodium? None of us, at least not in the concentrations to which we have become accustomed. And it *is* just a habit—you are not born with an appetite for salt; it is an acquired taste that can be unlearned. Now you may say, "I don't use a lot of salt on my food," or, "OK, I promise I'll cut down on salting my food." Although this will help lower your intake of sodium (and not using salt in cooking is a major prerequisite to all the Diet Principal diets, even the Diet for Life), unfortunately it's not enough, because many of the foods we are so used to eating already have an enormous sodium content. Did you add a teaspoon of salt to your veal stew recipe yesterday? That was 2196 mgs. of sodium right there. Had a Big Mac, lately? That's 1500 mgs of sodium in one fell swoop. How about ½ a cup of cottage cheese on your latest diet? 435 mgs. Did you have it with two celery stalks? That's another 250 mgs. of sodium.

Now I'm not trying to make you crazy with all this information about the dangers of over-sodiumizing your body. But if you want to lose weight, keep it off, and most important of all, stay healthy in the process, you have to know what's in

SODIUM CONTENT OF COMMON FOODS *

FOOD	AMOUNT	SODIUM (MGS)
Bacon		
Sliced	¼ pound	772
	2 slices	285
Canadian	¼ pound	2145
Beans		
Baked (canned)	1 cup	810
Green (canned)	1 cup	698
Bologna	¼ pound	1475
	2 slices	450
Bread		
Crumbs	½ cup	368
White	2 slices	234
Whole wheat	2 slices	214
Butter	¼ cup	560
Cheese		
American, grated	½ cup	350
Cottage	½ cup	435
American (processed)	1 ounce	238
Chicken (Kentucky Fried)	3 pieces	2285
Chili with beans	1 cup	1354
Corn, creamed (canned)	1 cup	604
Corn flakes	1¼ cup	320

FOOD	AMOUNT	SODIUM (MGS)
Corned beef	¼ pound	1474
Corned beef hash	1 cup	1188
Crab (canned)	1 cup	1600
Egg McMuffin	1	914
Ham, cured	¼ pound	854
Hamburger, Big Mac	1	1500
Hot Dog	2	1248
Hot dogs/beans (canned)	1 cup	958
Olives	2	312
Pickle, kosher dill	1	1000
Pie		
Apple	1 piece	482
Lemon meringue	1 piece	395
Pecan	1 piece	354
Pizza, frozen cheese	2 slices	925
Pork and beans (canned)	1 cup	1158
Potato chips	15	246
Pretzels	15	730
Pudding, bread w/raisins	1 cup	533
Rice, white, cooked w/ salt	1 cup	767
Salmon, canned pink	½ cup	426
Sauerkraut	1 cup	1755
Scallops	½ cup	578
Shrimp	½ cup	318
Soups, canned		
Bean and pork	1 cup	1008
Beef consomme	1 cup	782
Beef noodle	1 cup	1872
Cream of chicken	1 cup	970
Cream of potato	1 cup	1274
Chicken noodle	1 cup	979
Clam chowder, white	1 cup	938
Minestrone	1 cup	995
Onion	1 cup	1051
Tomato	1 cup	970
Vegetable beef	1 cup	1046
Soy sauce	1 tablespoon	1319
Tomato juice	1 cup	744
Turkey, white meat	¼ pound	93

* *Data compiled from chart appearing in John D. Kirschmann,* Nutritional Almanac Cookbook *(New York: McGraw Hill, 1983).*

what you eat; later, when you look at the Forbidden Foods chart on pages 82–85, you'll be able to spot *why* these foods are so dangerous to your health.

The chart on pages 54–55 lists a sample of foods and their sodium content.

Now, if the above list seems to you to be made up of everything you always wanted to eat but didn't have the time to, read the following list of foods low in sodium and you'll see how much "good" stuff is left for your enjoyment and your health. Foods low in sodium include: fruits; vegetables like broccoli, cauliflower, lettuce, mushrooms, potatoes, tomatoes; spinach, and squash; milk; flour; garlic; honey; jams; oils; pasta; popcorn; rice (cooked without salt); chicken; turkey; veal; lamb; and some others (see the complete chart of the nutritional contents of foods, pages 77–85).

One more thing—when reading the "foods with sodium" chart, remember that some of the foods that may seem high in sodium are not so bad when taken in smaller quantities. Thus the story of sodium is much like the story of other "things you don't need"—if you at least try to limit your intake, you'll be way ahead of the game of staying healthy. Here are some hints:

- Don't salt your food; re-educate your taste buds to enjoy food without added salt.

- Don't keep a salt shaker on your table—it's just extra temptation you don't need. If the shaker is not there, in time you'll forget all about it.

- Use herbs and spices instead of salt, or garlic, onions, or lemon juice for added flavor.

- Try substituting similar foods for those you are used to that contain a lot of sodium. For example, 8 unsalted peanuts have less than 1 mg. of sodium, while the same amount of salted peanuts has 35 mgs. Unsalted potato chips have 7 times less sodium (I am so used to eating these that the salted ones taste positively awful to me!). One-half cup of unsalted popcorn has almost no trace of sodium, while a cup of salted popcorn has over 150 mgs. You'll find that I use low-sodium Worcestershire sauce in my recipes—that's because one tablespoon has 3.5 mgs. of sodium, while one tablespoon of the regular kind has over 300 mgs. Quite a difference, right?

I'll take a risk here—I guarantee you that after a month of eating without salt, anything with sodium in it will taste *too* salty to you, and you will have won the battle. Believe me, it's easier than you think!

Caffeine

We're not even going to discuss chocolate. The fact that it contains sugar, the fact that one ounce of chocolate has about 10 mgs. of caffeine, and the fact that it is high in calories immediately qualify it as "forbidden" on the Diet to Lose and "OK once in a while" for the rest of your life. But you already knew that.

Now for coffee.

OK—you can keep the coffee. Drinking coffee in moderation seems to be fine for most people. But after you read some facts about overdosing on caffeine, you may at least want to reconsider and cut down from the four-cup-a-day habit.

And habit it is. Caffeine is an addictive drug, but one that is not always *that* harmful to your body. Explains Hermien Lee, "A small cup of coffee, about 6 ounces, can have a high concentration of caffeine, about 79–180 mgs., depending on whether you use brewed or instant. In many ways, coffee is wonderful. It is almost non-caloric (unless you drink it with a lot of sugar and cream), it is an effective stimulant that keeps you awake and can make you work at a more productive rate, and it tastes wonderful."

"But," continues Lee, "the fact remains that caffeine is an addictive drug, and like all drugs it has its drawbacks. This means that for some percentage of the population, drinking coffee has its hazards. One, it has been cited as aggravating cysts in women who are predisposed to developing them. Two, because it is absorbed into your body almost immediately, it causes your heart rate to increase, and this can mean trouble for some people. Three, it increases the secretion of acid in your stomach and is therefore a problem for people with any stomach disorders (it can cause severe heartburn)."

Below you'll find the caffeine content of those drinks that have certainly passed your lips at one time or another.

Caffeine is a natural diuretic, and that may account for its popularity among dieters. I have stayed away from coffee because I believe that the high concentration of caffeine is not great for the body. (You can drink decaffeinated coffee, but you should know that it still has some caffeine in it and is also

CAFFEINE IN COMMON DRINKS*

DRINK	AMOUNT	CAFFEINE (MGS)
Instant coffee	6-ounce cup	79
Brewed coffee	6-ounce cup	120–180
Decaffeinated	6-ounce cup	3
Tea (tea bag)	6-ounce cup	35–50
Iced tea		
Instant, lemon-flavored, no sugar	8-ounce cup	20–40
Home-made, lemon, no sugar	8-ounce cup	30–35
Coca Cola	12 ounces	35–65
Hot cocoa	6 ounces	10–20

* Data supplied by the American Tea Council

chemically processed.) Besides the problems noted above, studies are turning up everywhere showing that the caffeine found in coffee could be responsible for a myriad of diseases. For example, a 1984 study by doctors at Stanford University confirmed what similar European studies had already found, namely that there is a correlation between drinking a lot of coffee (more than 2 cups a day was considered to be "a lot") and developing a high level of cholesterol, and thereby heart disease.

Thus it seems that drinking less coffee or giving it up altogether can only be beneficial to your health. Instead of coffee I drink a lot of tea. In fact you'll find that all the Diet Principal food programs call for drinking at least 3–6 servings of hot or iced tea a day, specifically because we need all that liquid and tea has the added bonus of having little caffeine but enough to act as a diuretic.

But, you naturally ask, if I'm so high on tea, which contains some caffeine, why am I down on coffee? The answer to that is simple—most teas (excluding herb teas, which may not have caffeine but do have natural chemicals that can have an adverse effect on your system) contain much less caffeine than coffee, unless they are brewed to be as dark as coffee (that means steeping the tea bag or brewing the tea leaves for 3–5 minutes).

The rule is, when you prepare your *hot tea*, steep the tea bag for 15–30 seconds. That's plenty—you get the taste of tea and you get enough caffeine to help as a diuretic but not enough to really hurt you. If you use loose tea, put a teaspoon of the tea in a small tea-colander and pour hot water over it into a cup. Don't put the loose tea in the cup and let it brew—that will result in stronger tea, which you don't need. In both cases, add artificial sweetener and lemon, or nonfat or low-fat milk. The latter can compensate for the acidity that sometimes bothers some people; it also partially neutralizes the effects of the tannin in the tea, which can cause constipation.

For fresh *iced tea,* make the hot tea, pour it into a glass or pitcher, and add sliced lemon and a couple of slices of oranges (for an added treat—and extra vitamin C). You can add sweetener, if you like, but try the lemon and orange slices trick first —that should give the iced tea an added flavor so that you won't need sugar or sweetener. If you use instant iced tea, use the kind without sugar (you can add artificial sweetener, but no sugar). If you use a mix with lemon in it, you may still want to add lemon and orange slices (unless you have a problem with an acid stomach, in which case you might like to add low-fat or nonfat milk instead).

The point to remember is, if you follow the "moderation in everything" philosophy, you *can* drink some coffee, and if it is made right, you can drink as much tea as you like.

Alcohol

Will she leave us nothing? Actually, if you count up the "things you don't need," the list is not very long. Alcohol fits in here just fine, even though in moderation it is not harmful to your body (unless you are an alcoholic, in which case you need professional help for what is now recognized as a widespread disease). But you should be aware of the fact that, taken in large doses, alcohol drains your body of its minerals and deprives it of necessary vitamins, especially the B vitamins.

Moreover, if you are on a diet or want to maintain your weight, you'd better watch your intake of alcohol. Alcohol has no nutritional value whatsoever, and it is highly caloric—a can of beer has 175–200 calories ("light" beer still has about 95 calories), a 1½-ounce shot of vodka has 97–125 calories, an ounce of most liqueurs has 75–115 calories, and a glass of dry, table wine has 75–90 calories.

Thus, if you are not trying to lose weight, you may drink

alcohol in moderation without much worry for the calories you are taking in. This is true for all of us when we are on the Diet for Life, when a glass of wine or any other drink is not counterproductive or dangerous. (But always remember: never drink and drive!) When we are on the 30-Day Diet to Lose, however, any consumption of alcohol means we will take in empty calories that we don't need, and perhaps replace needed nutrients with these empty calories when we can least afford to do so.

Fast Foods

We may not nutritionally need fast foods, but on any day of the year one out of twelve Americans has eaten at McDonald's. A lunch consisting of a hamburger, french fries, and a milk shake totals about 950 calories. Since the government recommends a diet containing between 1200 and 2000 calories a day, the average "drive in and drive out, I'm in a terrible hurry" customer of a fast-food chain has consumed at least half his or her daily allotment of calories in one meal. If you eat breakfast, lunch, and dinner at fast-food restaurants, you are likely to consume almost 3000 calories a day, half of which come from our old enemy, fat. If you glance at the Contents of Fast Foods chart, you can also easily see that most of these are foods which lack vitamin A and C, are high in sodium and sugar, and are extremely high in saturated fat.*

Now, to try to break America of the fast-food habit would be useless, and somewhat unfair. These meals are affordable, they provide some people with the only protein they get during the day, their convenience makes life easier in a world that

* See Tom Davis, "Facts about Fast Food," *Consumer's Research Magazine*, Vol. 67, No. 8 (August 1984)

is already much too complicated, and we have to admit, they taste good.

The trick is to try to limit the foods you eat at these restaurants and balance them with nutritional meals at other times of the day. For example, if you just have to have that burger at the drive-in, go ahead and do it. But try to make dinner a vegetable and fruit affair so you can limit your intake of fat for the day. If you have eggs, bacon, hash brown potatoes, and buttered toast for a breakfast meeting on the run, have a salad for lunch.

CONTENTS OF FAST FOODS*

FOOD	CALORIES	FAT (GRAMS)	SODIUM (MGS)
Burrito, bean	350	10.8	1047
Chili dog	269	14	1000
Chili con carne	250	9.9	728
Cole slaw	118	8	256
Egg McMuffin	352	20	911
Fish sandwich	440	24	707
French fries	211	10.6	112
Fried chicken dinner	830	46.0	535 +
Fried shrimp, serving	381	24.4	537
Hamburger	290	13	525
Cheeseburger	350	17	724
Big Mac/Whopper	541–630	31–36	963
Hot dog	291	17	800
Milk shake			
Chocolate	324	8.4	329
Vanilla	324	7.8	250
Onion rings	300	17	N/A
Pizza (3 slices)	450	15.0	1140
Taco	186	9	79

* Chart data from Tom Davis, ''Facts about Fast Food,'' Consumer's Research Magazine, Vol. 67, No. 8 (August 1984), pp. 12–14; and Catherine F. Adams, Nutritive Value of American Foods, U.S. Dept. of Agriculture Handbook No. 456, Nov. 1975.

Opposite is a chart listing the nutritional contents (and non-contents) of some common "fast foods." Please read it so you will be more informed about what you're eating. Then, next time you order that Big Mac, at least you'll remember to go easy on dinner that night.

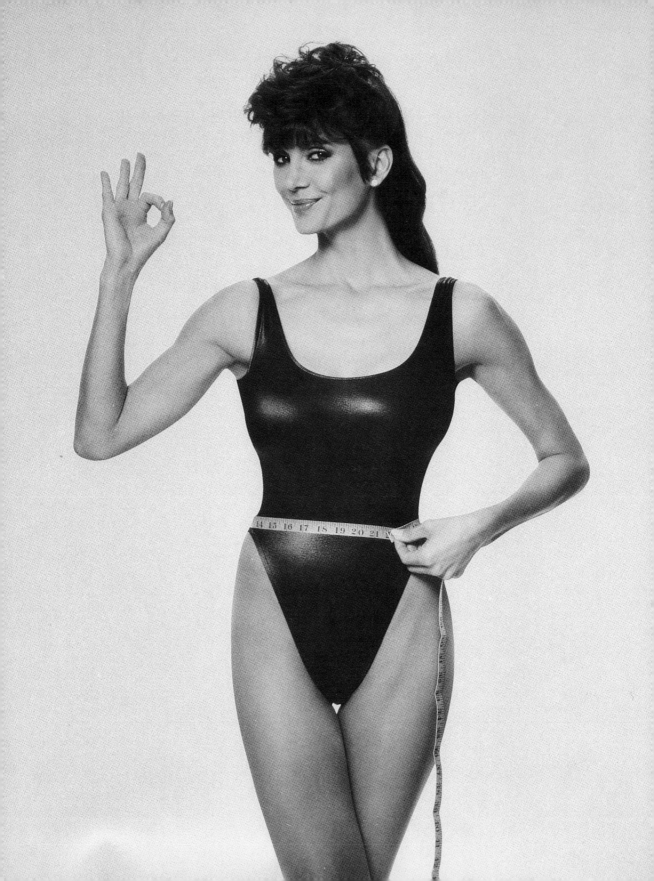

CHAPTER 3

THE 30-DAY DIET TO LOSE

When you're on your fifth diet of the year and you've done nothing but lose and gain, lose and gain, it seems as if every word you hear has to do with food. Everyone around you has a new suggestion about *the* diet that will surely work this time. Someone says to you, "If nothing else works, you can always try acupuncture—maybe you can make it 'leak' out and off." But it's not funny.

Nothing about the frustration of dieting is funny. Millions of Americans go on diets every week; millions more go off diets every week. For every person there is a diet that promises to work; for every person there are hundreds that don't. For every theory on food and on nutrition, there are experts who will agree with it and as many who will refute it. For every new courier who brings good news about the miracles of the diet of the week, there is yet another oracle who swears that just the opposite is true. It's enough to make you mad.

It did in my case. Throughout my life I had tried diet after diet. Most of the time I merely wanted to lose a few pounds. Sometimes I needed to lose more. Always I searched for the answer that would work once and for all, that would be permanent. And that's how the Diet Principles were born. After years of research, and trial and error, I have tried to condense it all into a program that works by providing a nutritious diet to help you lose weight successfully and permanently, and that introduces you to a way of eating that will keep you slim and healthy for the rest of your days. The Diet Principles will change your life.

The 30-Day Diet to Lose is just what it says—a sensible, successful way of eating that will help you to lose that extra weight safely and permanently. I have already discussed why we eat too much. I've explained what is in what we eat, why we are what we eat, and why we should eat some foods and avoid others. I have discussed the importance of moderation in eating, of balancing food so that you get enough of each nutrient your body needs to function properly, and of eating a variety of foods for a totally healthy body. Now, assuming that you have made the commitment to learn a new way of eating and have decided once and for all to lose that weight and keep it off, it is time to learn the principles of the 30-Day Diet to Lose.

THE PRINCIPLES

Think of these not really as rules, but as intelligent proposals it would be wise to follow. And don't be intimidated by their number—after a week it will seem as if you've always known them. After two weeks you'll wonder how you ever did without them. After a month you'll swear you knew them all along.

1. The 30-Day Diet to Lose has been nutritionally balanced to take into account the fact that you want to lose weight yet still need those daily requirements of nutrients so essential to your health. It contains a combination of foods which will supply you with these nutrients and also rid your body of extra, unwanted fat. However, I am not a doctor or a nutritionist. Although this diet has been undertaken by many "guinea pigs" (my co-workers and friends over the years) and has been examined by both the Food and Drug Administration and a nutritionist, I still urge you to see a doctor or a nutritionist before embarking on this (or any) diet. Every individual is unique—my body may react differently to a change in nutrition than yours will. That's why it is always a good idea to see a doctor before you begin.

2. The diet is a 30-day diet. Don't go on it for five days and then take a vacation. People who diet during the week and binge on weekends may as well forget the diet altogether. As Hermien Lee reminds us, "What will happen to the week dieter and weekend binger is that pretty soon the week goes from Monday to Wednesday and the weekend from Thursday to Monday." Need I say more?

3. The first week is the toughest. Don't get discouraged. Keep your goals in mind at all times. After the first week, you will have shrunk your stomach and won't miss food as much. Remember, you are not only eating less but are also eating differently in order to teach your body and mind a new and healthier way to eat. It takes a little time to get used to anything that's new, but it will be worth it. Just take it a day at a time. Think of the day you have just completed successfully, or the day you are about to start. But don't count the days that are left. Also, try to keep your mind off food. Thinking or talking about the diet you are on is boring to everyone, including yourself. Make the diet an ordinary part of your life, not an obsession. And no guilt, please—if you fall off, just get back on.

4. You should weigh yourself before embarking on the diet, just so you know how much weight you need to lose. Don't weigh yourself every morning, noon, and night. Not even every morning and night. Watch your body and not your scale, and you'll notice a difference without worrying about the pounds. Weigh yourself every other day, or every three days. When you do, make sure it is in the morning, about ten minutes after you get up, before you drink anything. And weigh yourself naked—for one thing, it's more accurate, and for another, looking at yourself naked is almost always guaranteed to spur you on to stay on the diet.

As for determining how much weight you should lose, that's a difficult question to answer. Weight charts found in magazines and doctors' offices never agree on how much you should weigh, and anyway I have found that the weight they suggest is much too high. Over the years I have collected such charts. One says that a 5'3" woman who is between twenty-five and thirty-four years old and has a medium frame should weigh between 116–130 pounds. That's a large span—and 130 is a lot of weight for a woman of that size. Another chart suggests that this woman should weigh between 108–120 pounds.

I believe that you yourself or your doctor can tell how much weight you need to lose. And be realistic in your assessment. Just because your best friend weighs 105 doesn't mean that is the best weight for you. Your doctor knows the characteristics of your health that may bear on your ideal weight. You yourself probably know at which weight you are most comfortable. Listen to both your doctor and yourself, and then embark on the diet.

5. Get a good night's sleep every night while you are on this diet. It is not unusual to be irritable and cranky when you are on a diet, especially during the first week. You may also be tired, and your moods may fluctuate. Getting a good night's sleep will alleviate much of this tension.

6. When was the last time you weighed your food to see how much you were eating? How about the last time you counted the amount of potassium or calcium you took that day? I have always refused to get into such a pattern of minutely measuring and accounting for everything I put into my mouth. It is time-consuming, it is difficult to accomplish well, and it is annoying. I have always felt that it is next to impossible to both enjoy myself and spend my time worrying about and enumerating the foods I eat. Thus *the Diet Principle of Principles is to follow the diet as closely as you can—and continue with your life.* I have already measured the amounts of food. I have already calculated the nutrients in each meal. All you have to do is re-educate yourself about the foods you should and should not eat, and follow the diet as planned.

7. This one is hard—maybe the hardest. Learn control! Commitment is one thing, but it has to be followed by control so you can stick to your commitment. The best way I have found to control what I eat is to first make a list of those foods I can't get enough of (or can't "control"), and make them "forbidden" until they take on less importance in my life. When I stopped eating cheese, I stopped cold turkey. Not even a slice of pizza crossed my lips, because I knew if I ate one bite I wouldn't be able to stop. Explains Hermien Lee, "When people eat pizza, they don't think about their body or about being overweight. It's only when they're through eating that pizza that they think about being fat." So think about it before you begin. And if you can't control eating chocolate, don't eat it at all until you develop that control. Take some satisfaction and pride in having that control, and be secure in the knowledge that after a short time you won't even miss that food you so crave.

8. You can be well fed and not well nourished. What does this mean? Some diets insist that you count calories. I don't, mainly because counting calories does not ensure proper nutrition. For example, if your daily calorie allowance is 1500 and you eat an apple pie with melted cheese and two malted milks, you'll fulfill your calorie allowance but you'll get a far-from-nourishing meal. Just eat the meals as prescribed and don't worry about counting calories.

9. Drink a glass of water or iced tea (see rule on p. 59 on how to make tea) before each meal, preferably 15–20 minutes before. You'll get the fluid your body needs, and you'll fill up your stomach so you'll be less inclined to overeat. Before you start on the diet, buy yourself a beautiful 8-ounce glass. When you are at home, serve yourself the water or iced tea in this special glass. If you have an office, get yourself a glass to keep there. It will be a constant reminder of how thirsty you should be and of how much weight you are losing. I have found that this makes the drinking a classy event and not a minor annoyance.

10. Eat the foods listed in the combinations prescribed. Don't switch meals. You can substitute one day for another *if you must*, but I'd prefer you to stick to the diet as closely as possible (especially for the first week, when the weight loss is the greatest). I have found that these food combinations work well together in your system, both to provide you with the nutrients you need and at the same time to reduce your weight.

11. Don't eat and watch television at the same time. Actually, don't eat and do anything else at the same time. If you are distracted, you will probably eat more than you should. If you concentrate on eating and are aware of what you are putting into your mouth, chances are you will eat less.

12. Serve your meals on attractive salad plates (or small dinner plates). First of all, a pretty table will make you smile, and that's a good way to begin enjoying your meal (even if you are eating less than you are used to). Besides, just because you are on a diet doesn't mean you have to eat on paper plates. Second, common sense would tell you that putting smaller portions on smaller plates makes the portions seem bigger (or at least not as tiny).

13. Eat only in the kitchen or in the dining room—in other words, in places that are meant for eating.

14. Try to develop your own little tricks to lessen your intake of certain foods. For example:

- Whenever you eat a salad, ask for the dressing on the side and leave it there. Before each bite, dip the fork into the dressing and then take a bite of the salad (you'll get the taste of the dressing but use much less).

- Chew your food longer—you won't put as much food into your mouth because you'll be too busy chewing what's already there. (You'll also find that you taste your food more and thus enjoy it more.)

15. Never, ever eat after eight o'clock at night while on this diet. (This is a good rule to follow at all times, but it is really necessary on this diet.) The food you eat after eight will just sit in your stomach. And just think how much time you'll have left over to do other things!

16. Chicken makes up a large part of this diet. Learn the recipes and follow them closely. Don't substitute butter for margarine; don't use salt when it's not called for; and don't leave the skin on the chicken (taking it off will cut your intake of fat and cholesterol by as much as one-half!). Try to buy chicken that has not been treated with hormones (the reason some farmers give their chickens hormones is to make them fatter; since your aim is *not* to get fatter, try to buy other chickens).

17. On this diet you are allowed an occasional egg, for the protein. If you have a problem with cholesterol (as diagnosed by your doctor, not by your mother), ask your doctor if you can eat the eggs. If not, you can substitute egg whites and leave out the yellow (that's the part with the cholesterol). Try making an omelet using the whites of two eggs, salsa (a Mexican condiment made of tomatoes, peppers, and onions—see page 184 for recipe), and some onions. Or you can hard-boil an egg, discard the yolk, slice the white, and eat that with the tomatoes and toast.

18. When the diet calls for toast, make it whole wheat for the extra fiber. And don't think you are doing yourself a favor by skipping the toast. If the menu says to eat it, then eat it!

19. Take a multivitamin and calcium supplement. As you know from reading the section on calcium in Chapter II (see page 34), we need at least 1200–1500 mgs. of calcium every day. Since this diet is low in dairy products (a good source of calcium but also a high source of fat), you need to eat those vegetables that contain calcium (see the food chart for added information) and still take a supplement every day. Ask your doctor which supplement he or she prefers. A calcium pill a day will go a long way toward ensuring that you get your daily supply.

20. Not a canned product shall you open during the thirty days—not a soup, not a tomato sauce, not a canned peach. Tuna or salmon packed in water are fine, but that's it. If you read Chapter III, you already know that canned foods often contain too much sodium, sugar, and oil. Leave them sealed on the shelf, or use them for door stops.

21. Some breakfasts call for cereal. Read the cereal box before you buy it. Almost all cereals contain an unnecessarily high amount of sugar and sodium. Even the so-called granolas are not terrific. I eat Cheerios because it is low in sugar and sodium, but there are other grain cereals which are also nutritious.

22. Salads taste better with dressings—we all figured that out a long time ago. Follow the salad fork hint, and do it with low-cal dressings. Leave out the "cream" salad dressings. Your body doesn't need anything that's in them. One of my favorite dressings is made by combining Japanese rice vinegar with Dijon mustard (see No-Guilt Salad Dressing, page 180).

23. Pasta is on this diet, and it is good for you. But don't add oil or salt to the water. When the pasta is done, be sure to rinse it in cold water to get rid of the extra starch.

24. The best thing to drink on this diet is iced tea or water. However, if you just can't live without colas and the like, at least make them "diet" drinks.

25. If you find that you need extra nourishment during the day, eat an apple, an orange, a teaspoon of peanut butter (the one without oil—for Hermien Lee's recipe, see page 218), but never a chocolate bar. Remember, you are going to lose weight. Save the chocolate bar, if you must, for an occasional diversion from the Diet for Life.

26. I don't use salt on anything. If you must have it, use a salt substitute. But the better road to take is to forget the salt (you won't miss it—after a while you won't even like it anymore!). Learn to use other spices to please your taste buds. I put garlic on anything that will let me (if you get garlic breath, an antacid will neutralize the acid in your stomach and reduce the odor). Those seasonings that I use liberally include:

Basil	Garlic powder	Orange bits
Celery powder	(not salt)	Oregano
(not salt)	Ginger	Parmesan cheese
Cinnamon	Italian herb mixture	(grated)
Cloves	(good on spaghetti	Pepper (red, black,
Curry	sauce and salads)	and white)
Dill	Lemon bits	Poppy seeds
Dry mustard	Nutmeg	Sage
		Sesame seeds

27. There's no point to dieting if you are not going to exercise. As you lose weight, you need to tone your body in order to avoid flabbiness. However, if you have not exercised in some time before going on the diet, I realize that it is difficult enough to go on a diet, without starting yet another regimen like exercising. I would advise you at least to do some isometric exercises (see *The Body Principal*), which are not difficult, not time-consuming, and will help in toning your body and getting you back into shape.

THE "PERFECT FOODS"

You may think that nothing is perfect, but some foods are. The "Perfect Foods" have all the vitamins and minerals your body needs and none of those "bad" things it doesn't need. All these foods are on the 30-Day Diet to Lose, but obviously they can and should be eaten anytime. Read the list starting on page 76 and then try to remember them; whenever the chance comes up to eat something on this list, do it! You'll be doing yourself a great favor.

THE "(ALMOST ALWAYS) FORBIDDEN FOODS"

There are some foods I never eat. Well, almost never. Since I've already said that I don't believe in total denial, I'd better explain that the title "(Almost Always) Forbidden Foods" means that these foods are not good for you and you shouldn't make eating any of them a habit. But if you want an anchovy once a month, eat it. Don't feel guilty—just eat it! At least you will have made an informed decision, knowing full well what is in what you are eating.

We've already talked about salt (see Chapter II, page 53). Then there is cheese. In *The Body Principal* I made the point that I never eat cheese because it is concentrated fat. "If you insist on eating it, you might as well spread it on your thighs, because that's where it will surely show up anyway, sooner than later." I still hold fast to that belief, and although many people believe that low-fat cheese is acceptable, I feel that no cheese is best.

The question of margarine vs. butter is still being debated not only in households everywhere but by nutritionists and food writers. Butter has fat and cholesterol, while margarine, although unsaturated and low in cholesterol (some brands have none at all), is a processed food and contains chemicals. My feeling is, when your aim is to lose weight you should not use butter and should use only a minimum amount of margarine. After that, it's up to you—but always try to use only a small amount.

As for mayonnaise—forget it. It is full of fat and salt. If you want to use it, put it on your face to add oil to your skin. I substitute nonfat plain yogurt for mayonnaise in recipes and have as yet had no complaints.

The following charts—The Perfect Foods, The Maybe/Sometimes Foods, and The (Almost Always) Forbidden Foods—list the nutritional contents of these foods. They are for informational purposes, so that when you are preparing the various recipes, or when you eat food that you have not prepared, you will know what's in what you eat.

PERFECT FOODS

FOOD	WHAT IT HAS
Dried Beans and Peas (Legumes)	Protein Fiber Vitamin B_2, B_3 Potassium Iron Low in fat
Bread and cereal (Whole wheat)	Protein Complex carbohydrates Fiber Vitamin B Low in fat No cholesterol
Chicken and turkey	Protein Low in fat
Fish (Not canned in oil; no lobster; small amounts of shrimp; salmon, flounder, sole, and other white fish are great)	Protein Low in fat, cholesterol, calories
Fruits	All vitamins
Nonfat Yogurt/Milk	Protein Vitamin A Vitamin B_1, B_2, B_6, B_{12} Vitamin D Magnesium Calcium Low in sodium, fat, calories
Vegetables	Complex carbohydrates Fiber Vitamin A Vitamin C Calcium Low in fat, calories No cholesterol

THE CONTENTS OF FOOD—THE PERFECT FOODS

Food	Amt	Calor	Pro (gms)	Fat (gms)	Carb (gms)	MINERALS Calc. (mgs)	Pho (mgs)	Iro (mgs)	Sod (mgs)	Pot (mgs)	VITAMINS A (IU)	C (mgs)
Beans												
Kidney	1 cup	218	14.4	.9	39.6	70	259	4.4	6	629	10	
Green, cooked	1 cup	31	2	.3	6.8	63	46	.8	5	189	680	15
Lentil	1 cup	212	15.6		38.6	50	238	4.2		498	40	
Bread, whole wheat	1 slice	56	2.4	.7	11	23	52	.5	121	63		
Cereal												
Bran flakes	1 cup	106	3.6	.6	28.2	19	125	12.4	207	137	1650	12
Cheerios												
Chicken												
Breast	½ pound	198	37.3	9		20	384	2.2	189	815	135	5.7
Leg	½ pound	157	26	15		18	253	2.2	189	815	170	6
Thigh	½ pound	218	30.8	16.8		20	317	2.7	189	815		
Milk, nonfat	1 cup	86	8.4	.4	11.8	302	247	.1	126	406	500	2.4
Fish												
Bass	½ pound	236	42.9	4.8			436		154	580		4.5
Cod	½ pound	177	39.9	1.7		23	440	.9	159	866		
Halibut	½ pound	227	47.4	2.5		30	479	1.6	122	1019	2000	
Salmon, canned	1 cup	310	45.1	13		431	629	1.8	851	794	150	5.2
Snapper	½ pound	211	44.9	2.7		37	486	1.8	152	733		
Tuna, canned W	1 cup	254	56	1.6		32	380	3.2	82	558		4.4
Flour, whole wheat	½ cup	200	5.8	.6	41.9	53	48	.4	1	53		

THE CONTENTS OF FOOD—THE PERFECT FOODS (continued)

Food	Amt	Calor	Pro (gms)	Fat (gms)	Carb (gms)	MINERALS					VITAMINS	
						Calc (mgs)	Pho (mgs)	Iro (mgs)	Sod (mgs)	Pot (mgs)	A (IU)	C (mgs)
Fruit												
Apple	1	96	.3	1	24	12	17	.5	2	181	150	7
Applesauce	1 cup	100	.5	.5	26.4	10	12	1.2	5	190		
Apricot, dried	½ cup	169	3.3	.4	43.3	44	70	3.6	17	637	7085	8
Banana	1	127	1.6	.3	33.3	12	39	1	2	550		
Blueberries	1 cup	90	1	.7	22.2	22	19	1.5	1	117		
Cantaloupe	¼	30	.7	.1	7.3	32	30	2	1	193		
Dates	5	137	1.1	.2	36.5	30	32	1.5		324		
Grapes	1 cup	106	2	1.5	24	24	18	.6	5	242		
Orange	1	64	1.3	.3	16	54	26	.5	1	263		
Papaya	½	58	.9		15	30	20	.5	5	351		
Peach	1	38	.6		9.7	9	19	.5	1	202		
Pear	1	122	1.4	.8	30.6	16	22	.6	4	260		
Strawberries	1 cup	56	1	.8	12.6	32	32	1.5	2	246		
Lettuce												
Bibb	1 cup	8	.7		1.4	19	14	1	5	145	530	4
Red leaf	1 cup	10	.7	.2	1.9	37	14	.8	5	145	1050	10
Bran muffin	1	104	3.1	3.9	17.2	57	162	1.5	179	172	90	
Parmesan, grated	1 Tbs	23	2	1.5	.2	69	40	.05	93	5	35	
Popcorn, plain	1 cup	54	1.8	.7	10.7	2	39	.4		34		
Potato, baked	1	145	4		32	14	101	1	6	782		
Rice, brown, cooked	1 cup	178	3.8	1.2	38.2	18	110	.8	423	105		31
Spaghetti	1 cup	155	4.8	.6	32.2	11	70	1.3		85		

Food	Amount											
Tea, light	1 cup	4	.1		.9	5	4	.2		58		
Tortilla	1 6"	63	1.5	.6	13.5	60	42	.9				
Turkey	½ pound	399	75	8.9		18	481	2.7	186	932		
Veal cutlet	¼ pound	170	18.1	10.1		10.3	184	2.7	63	289		
Vegetables												
Artichoke	1	44	2.8	.2	9.9	51	69	1.1	30	301	150	8
Asparagus	1 cup	35	3.4	.3	6.8	30	84	1.4	3	375	1220	45
Broccoli, cooked	1 cup	40	4.8	.5	70	136	96	1.2	16	414	3800	140
Brussels sprouts	1	56	6.5	.6	10	50	112	1.7	16	423	810	2
Carrots, cooked	1 cup	48	1.4	.3	11	37	36	.7	47	341	15750	17
Corn, cooked	1 cup	137	5.3	1.7	31	5	147	1		272	660	12
Cucumbers	1 cup	16	.9		3.6	26	28	1.2	6	168	260	12
Garlic	1 clove	4	.2		.9	23	36	2.1	6	264		4
Spinach, cooked	1 cup	41	5.4		6.5	167	68	4	90	583	14580	50
Squash, summer, cooked	1 cup	25	1.6	.2	5.5		45	.7	2	254	700	18
Sweet potato, baked	1	161	2.4	.6	3	46	66	1	14	342	9230	25
Tomato, raw	1	33	1.6	.3	7	29	40	.8	4	366	1350	34
Wheat germ	½ cup	181	13.3	5	23.4	36	559	4.7		414	16	7
Yogurt, nonfat plain	1 cup	127	13	.4	17.4	452	355	.2	174	579		2

THE CONTENTS OF FOOD—THE MAYBE/SOMETIMES FOODS

Food	Amt	Calor	Pro (gms)	Fat (gms)	Carb (gms)	Calc (mgs)	Pho (mgs)	Iro (mgs)	Sod (mgs)	Pot (mgs)	A (IU)	C (mgs)
						MINERALS					VITAMINS	
Beer	12 ounces	150	1		14	18	108		25	90		
Canadian bacon	1 slice	58	5.7	3.7		3	46		537	91		
Cookies												
Chocolate Chip	4	205	2	12	24	14	40	.8	139	47	40	
Dough, plain	1	100	1	5	13	10	48	.4	125	23	20	
Fig Bars	4	200	2	3	42	44	34	1	141	111	60	
Oatmeal/Raisin	4	235	3	8	38	11	53	1.4	84	192	30	
Vanilla Wafers	10	185	2	6	30	16	25	.6	101	29	50	
Cranberry sauce	1 cup	405		1	104	17	11	.6	3	83	60	
Eggs												
Fried	1	85	5	6	1	26	80	.9	155	58	290	
Boiled	1	80	6	6	1	28	90	1.0	61	65	260	
Hard	1	80	6	6	1	28	90	1.0	61	65	260	
Scrambled	1	95	6	7	1	47	97	.9	164	85	310	
Oils												
Butter, unsalted	1 Tbs	100		12	[Chol: 31]	3	3		2	4	430	
Butter, whipped	1 Tbs	65		8		2	2		93	2	290	
Margarine, unsalted	1 Tbs	100		12	[Chol: 0]	3	3		1	4	470	
Margarine, soft	1 Tbs	100		12		3	3		140	4	470	

THE CONTENTS OF FOOD—THE MAYBE/SOMETIMES FOODS

Mayonnaise, low-fat	1 Tbs	20	2	2	3	4	19	1	40
Raisins									
Salad dressing									
Italian, low-cal	1 Tbs	10	1	2	1	118	2		
French, low-cal	1 Tbs	15	1	2	2	126	13		

THE CONTENTS OF FOOD—THE (ALMOST ALWAYS) FORBIDDEN FOODS

Food	Amt	Calor	Pro (gms)	Fat (gms)	Carb (gms)	MINERALS					VITAMINS	
						Calc (mgs)	Pho (mgs)	Iro (mgs)	Sod (mgs)	Pot (mgs)	A (IU)	C (mgs)
Anchovies	1 Tbl	42	21	2.3	1.4		20	25	2058			
Avocados	1	334	4	32.8	12.6	20	84	1	8	1208	580	28
Bacon	slice	1508	19	157	2.3	29	245	3	1542	295		
Baking soda	1 tsp								1123			
BBQ sauce	1 Tbl	14		1	1.3	3	3		127	27	56	1
Beef												
Corned	½ pound	665	36	56.5		21	283.5	5	2949	136		
Rump roast	1 pound	1167	67	97.4		39	616	10	235	1072	190	
T-steak	½ pound	798	29	84		16	271		104	473	150	
Candy, chocolate	1 ounce	147	2	9.2	16	65	65		27	109	80	
Cereals, sugared*												
Total	1 cup	109	3	1.0	22.7	39			412			
Life	1 cup	159	8	.8	29.1	147			237			
Cocoa Crispies	1 cup	106	1.4	.5	25.2	10			199			
Raisin Bran	1 cup	130	3.5	.5	40	35			194			
Corn Flakes	1 cup	110	2	1	23.7				251			
Granola	1 cup	128	3	4	18.8							
Cheese												
Blue	1 ounce	103	6	8.2		150	110		396	73	204	

Food	Amount										
Cheddar	1 ounce	112	7	9.4		211	145		176	28	300
Cottage, creamed	1 cup	217	26	9.5	5.6	126	277		850	177	342
Cream	1 ounce	105	2	10.6	.6	17	23		70	21	430
Processed American	1 ounce	107	7	8.9	.5	174	216		406	46	340
Swiss	1 ounce	107	8	7.8	1.0	31	171	.3	74	31	240
Drinks											
Colas	12 ounces	145			37						
Cream soda	12 ounces	160			40.8						
Root beer	12 ounces	150			39						
Meats											
Bologna	¼ pound	345	13	33	1.3	8	45	2	1474	260	
Ham, cured	¼ pound	384	17	34.5	5	9	101	2	854	267	
Hot dog	1	182	7	17.1	1	3	57		618		
Pork chop	¼ pound	286	16	24.2		9	142		86	255	
Salami	1 slice	90	5	7		3	57		353		
Sausage	1	70	3	6		3			125		
Milk											
Condensed	1 cup	980	24	27	166	868	775		343	1136	1000
Cream	1 Tbl	30	3	3	1	14	12		6	18	110

THE CONTENTS OF FOOD—THE (ALMOST ALWAYS) FORBIDDEN FOODS (continued)

Food	Amt	Calor	Pro (gms)	Fat (gms)	Carb (gms)	MINERALS					VITAMINS	
						Calc (mgs)	Pho (mgs)	Iro (mgs)	Sod (mgs)	Pot (mgs)	A (IU)	C (mgs)
Custard	½ cup	130	7	6	15	193	155		104	194	465	
Egg Nog	1 cup	340	10	19	34	330	278		312	420	890	
Evaporated	1 cup	340	17	19	25	657	510		297	764	610	
Ice Cream	1 cup	350	4	24	32	151	115		49	221	900	
Malted, Chocolate	1 cup	235	11	10	29	347	307		214	500	330	
Shake, Vanilla	1 cup	350	12	9	56	457	361			572	360	
Sour cream	1 cup	493	7	48.7	10	268	195		123	331	1817	
Whipped cream	1 cup	821	5	88	6.6	154	149		89	179	3499	
Oils												
Corn	1 Tbl	120										
Lard	1 Tbl	115										
Mayo	1 Tbl	101										
Olive	1 Tbl	120										
Peanut	1 Tbl	120										
Safflower	1 Tbl	120										
Olives, green	10	33		3.6		17	5	.5	686	16	90	
Peanut butter	1 Tbl	95	4	8	3	9	61	.3	97	100		

Food	Serving											
Pickles, dill	1	11		.4	2.2	26	21	1	1428	200	100	6
Pizza												
Cheese	3 slices	450	25	15	54	450			1350		750	
Pepperoni	3 slices	430	23	17	45	300			1500		1000	
Rice, white	1 cup	225	4		50	21	57	1.8	767	57		
Salt	1 tsp								2196			
Sauerkraut	1 cup	42	2	.5	9.4	85	42	1.2	1755	329	120	33
Snacks												
Potato chips												
w/salt	10	113	1.1	8	10	8	28	.4	sod?	226		3
Pretzels	10 twist	235	6	3	46	79			1008	78		
Soy sauce	1 Tbl	12	1	.2	1.7	15	19	15	1319	66		
Sweets												
Cream Pies												
Custard	1 slice	285	8	14	30	125	147	1.2	436	178	300	
Cherry	1 slice	412	4	18	61	22	40	.5	480	166	690	
Brown Sugar	1 cup	820			212	187	42	7.5	66	757		
White Sugar	1 cup	770			199				2	6		
	1 Tbl	45			12							

These cereals contain a lot more sugar than you would think. Just look at their sugar contents—Total: 8.3 percent; Life: 16 percent; Cocoa Crispies: 43 percent; Raisin Bran: 29 percent; Granola: 5.3 percent. Chart data compiled from John D. Kirschmann, Nutrition Almanac Cookbook (New York: McGraw Hill, 1983).

THE 30-DAY DIET TO LOSE

Basic Beverage Rule: 1 glass of water or iced tea, or cup of hot tea, before each meal, then one after the meal; drink an additional 2 glasses or cups any other time during the day. This will bring your total to 8 glasses of liquid every day. Remember, the tea should be light to minimize your intake of caffeine (see p. 59 for rule on how to make tea). You can, if you like, use iced-tea mix but make sure it doesn't contain either sugar or lemon. While sugar and cream are forbidden, nonfat milk may be added. This is an easy way to flush out your system and ensure your intake of 8 glasses of liquid every day.

BREAKFAST	LUNCH	DINNER
DAY 1		
Cereal with strawberries, nonfat milk	Spinach–Mushroom Salad (p. 110)	Baked Fillet of Sole (p. 103)
Hot tea or decaf	1 slice turkey, white meat	½ cup brown rice
Glass of water	2 melba toasts or low-sodium crackers	Steamed broccoli
	Beverage	Beverage
DAY 2		
1 egg, poached or boiled	Vegetable Salad (p. 109)	Broiled Marinated Chicken (p. 93)
1 slice wheat toast, dry	2 crackers or melba toasts	Half a boiled potato
2 slices tomato	Beverage	Steamed squash or spinach
Hot tea or decaf		Melba toast
		Beverage
DAY 3		
1 cup nonfat plain yogurt with ½ apple and ½ banana	1 slice wheat toast, dry, with lettuce and ½ cup water-packed tuna (cucumber slices, optional)	Steamed Vegetable Plate (p. 107)
Hot tea or decaf		Tomato Dressing (p. 116)
Glass of water	Beverage	2 slices wheat toast, dry
		Beverage

BREAKFAST	LUNCH	DINNER
DAY 4		
1 cup bran flakes with blueberries (if frozen, unsweetened), ½ cup nonfat milk Hot tea or decaf	Chicken Salad (p. 97) with low-cal dressing Beverage	Pasta with Vegetables Green lettuce salad Beverage
DAY 5		
1 slice melon ½ cup nonfat plain yogurt 1 slice Banana Bread (p. 114) Hot tea or decaf	Garden Green Salad (p. 111) 2 melba toasts Beverage	Broiled Herb/Garlic Chicken (p. 92) Steamed broccoli Beverage
DAY 6		
2 Salt-free rice cakes with low-cal jam 1 cup berries in bowl Hot tea or decaf	Salade Niçoise (p. 105) 2 breadsticks or 1 slice toast, dry Beverage	Steamed Vegetable Plate (p. 107) with grated Parmesan Beverage
DAY 7		
Mini Omelette (p. 112) 1 slice wheat toast, dry ½ orange Hot tea or decaf	Garden Green Salad, no tomato (p. 111) 1 melba toast	Fish–Broccoli Rolls in Wine Sauce (p. 102) Sliced Tomato Salad (p. 112) Beverage
DAY 8		
1 slice wheat toast, dry 1 slice melon Hot tea or decaf	Chinese-Sesame Chicken Salad (p. 98) Beverage	Steamed Vegetable Plate (p. 107) with grated Parmesan 2 breadsticks Beverage
DAY 9		
1 egg, poached 1 glass prune juice 1 slice wheat toast, dry Hot tea or decaf	Spinach– Mushroom Salad (p. 110) with low-cal dressing Beverage	Broiled Fresh Salmon Steaks (p. 99) ½ cup brown rice Sliced Tomato Salad (p. 112), no dressing Beverage

BREAKFAST	LUNCH	DINNER
DAY 10 Cereal with strawberries, ½ cup nonfat milk Hot tea or decaf	1 slice wheat toast, dry, with lettuce and 1 or 2 slices of turkey with low-cal dressing (open-face sandwich) Beverage	Steamed Vegetable Plate (p. 107) Beverage
DAY 11 1 cup nonfat plain yogurt, ½ apple, ½ banana Hot tea or decaf	Garden Green Salad (p. 111) 1 slice wheat toast or melba toast Beverage	Steamed Snapper with Scallions and Ginger (p. 100) ½ cup brown rice Steamed green beans Beverage
DAY 12 ½ melon 1 rice cake, low-cal jam Hot tea or decaf	Broiled Fish or Chicken (pp. 93 and 99) Garden Green Salad (p. 111) with low-cal dressing Beverage	Steamed Vegetable Plate (p. 107) Tomato Dressing (p. 116), optional Beverage
DAY 13 Cereal with fruit and ½ cup nonfat milk Hot tea or decaf	Spinach–Mushroom Salad (p. 110) Beverage	2 slices chicken, white meat 2 melba toasts Sliced Tomato Salad (p. 112) with dressing Steamed broccoli Beverage
DAY 14 Mini Omelette (p. 112) 1 slice wheat toast, dry 2 slices tomato Hot tea or decaf	Steamed Vegetable Plate (p. 107) 2 melba toasts Beverage	Baked or Broiled Fish with Dill (p. 103) ½ boiled potato Steamed green beans Beverage

BREAKFAST	LUNCH	DINNER
DAY 15 1 cup nonfat plain yogurt with ½ apple, ½ banana Hot tea or decaf	Four-Shrimp Salad (p. 104) with lettuce and low-cal dressing 2 melba toasts Beverage	Pasta with Vegetables (p. 188) 2 breadsticks Beverage
DAY 16 ½ cup bran flakes with berries and ½ cup nonfat milk Hot tea or decaf	Steamed Vegetable Plate (p. 107) 2 melba toasts Beverage	Chicken with Fried Onions (p. 94) Green lettuce salad Beverage
DAY 17 ½ melon with strawberries 2 melba toasts Hot tea or decaf	Garden Green Salad (p. 111) 2 melba toasts Beverage	Baked or Broiled Fish with Dill (p. 103) Sliced Tomato Salad (p. 112) with low-cal dressing Beverage
DAY 18 1 slice wheat toast, dry 4 slices tomato Hot tea or decaf	Salade Niçoise (p. 105) 2 breadsticks Beverage	Steamed Vegetable Plate (p. 107) Beverage
DAY 19 ½ cup nonfat plain yogurt 1 slice Banana Bread (p. 114) ½ apple, sliced Hot tea or decaf	Vegetable Salad (p. 109) with low-cal dressing 2 melba toasts Beverage	Chicken Kabobs (p. 96) ½ cup brown rice Beverage
DAY 20 1 glass prune juice Cereal with ½ cup nonfat milk Hot tea or decaf	Open-face Tuna Salad (p. 104) sandwich with tomato Beverage	Steamed Vegetable Plate (p. 107) Beverage

BREAKFAST	LUNCH	DINNER
DAY 21		
½ cup nonfat plain yogurt with ½ cup each of melon, strawberries, and bananas	Four-Shrimp Salad (p. 104) with lettuce	Curried Chicken (p. 95) ½ cup brown rice
Hot tea or decaf	2 melba toasts Beverage	Broiled Tomato Halves with Garlic (p. 108) Beverage
DAY 22		
Eggs Florentine (p. 113)	Steamed Vegetable Plate (p. 107)	Steamed Snapper with Scallions and Ginger (p. 100)
1 slice dry toast Hot tea or decaf	with grated Parmesan Beverage	½ cup brown rice Sliced Tomato Salad (p. 112) Beverage
DAY 23		
1 slice Banana Bread (p. 114)	Spinach– Mushroom Salad (p. 110)	Broiled Herb–Garlic Chicken or Turkey (p. 92)
1 slice melon Hot tea or decaf	Beverage	Garden Green Salad (p. 111) with low-cal dressing 2 melba toasts Beverage
DAY 24		
1 glass prune juice Cereal with ½ cup nonfat milk	Chicken Salad (p. 97) with tomato	Fish Kabobs (p. 101) ½ cup brown rice
1 slice melon Hot tea or decaf	2 melba toasts Beverage	Beverage
DAY 25		
2 rice cakes with low-cal jam	Italian Vegetable Salad (p. 110)	Pasta with Vegetables (p. 188)
1 slice melon Hot tea or decaf	2 breadsticks Beverage	Garden Green Salad (p. 111) with low-cal dressing Beverage

BREAKFAST	LUNCH	DINNER
DAY 26		
1 slice Banana Bread (p. 114)	Open-face Tuna Salad (p. 104) sandwich on wheat toast	Steamed Vegetable Plate (p. 107) with grated Parmesan
½ cup nonfat plain yogurt with ½ apple	1 slice tomato	Beverage
Hot tea or decaf	Beverage	
DAY 27		
Puffed rice cereal with strawberries	Spinach– Mushroom Salad (p. 110)	Broiled Herb– Garlic Chicken (p. 92)
½ cup nonfat milk	2 melba toasts	Steamed carrots and broccoli
Hot tea or decaf	Beverage	Beverage
DAY 28		
1 slice wheat toast, dry	Italian Vegetable Salad (p. 110)	Baked or Broiled Fish with Dill (p. 103)
1 slice melon	Beverage	Garden Green Salad (p. 111)
Hot tea or decaf		Beverage
DAY 29		
½ cup nonfat plain yogurt, ½ banana, ½ apple	Tuna Salad (p. 104)	Baked sweet potato
	Sliced tomato	Green lettuce salad
	2 breadsticks	Beverage
Hot tea or decaf	Beverage	
DAY 30		
Cereal with strawberries, ½ cup nonfat milk	Garden Green Salad (p. 111)	Harry Alan Salmon (p. 100)
	1 melba toast	½ cup brown rice
Hot tea or decaf	Beverage	Steamed broccoli
		Beverage

THE 30-DAY DIET TO LOSE RECIPES

The 30-Day Diet to Lose works. It works quickly, easily, healthfully. But as with any diet, sticking to the program is the key. And the reward is the best gift you could give yourself —when you finish the 30 days you will have lost the weight, and your new way of eating will ensure that you never put it back on.

Now for the recipes.

I love to cook and I have been collecting recipes for years. The recipes listed here are organized by food group. They are straightforward and self-explanatory, and they comprise all the dishes listed in this diet. (In Chapter IV you will find an additional 100 recipes that I have used on the Diet for Life).

CHICKEN

Broiled Herb–Garlic Chicken

    1 2-pound broiler chicken, quartered and skinned
2–3 garlic cloves, pressed
    Freshly ground black pepper to taste
½ teaspoon dried tarragon
1 cup hot water
2 tablespoons unsalted margarine
2 tablespoons chopped fresh parsley

Preheat oven to "Broil."

Skin the chicken and rub the meat well with the pressed garlic. When done, save the garlic. Put the chicken in a broiling pan and brown quickly on both sides under the preheated broiler (about 5 minutes on each side).

When browned, remove chicken and lower oven to 350°. Place the chicken in a baking dish and season with pepper, tarragon, and the garlic you used to rub the chicken. Bake in the 350° oven for about 20 minutes. In a small bowl, mix the hot water, margarine, and parsley, and use the mixture to baste the chicken while it is baking. Check periodically to see that it doesn't dry out. Serve with steamed broccoli and brown rice. SERVES 4

Note: You can refrigerate the leftover chicken to eat cold or for later use in Chicken Salad (see page 97).

Broiled Marinated Chicken

    6–8 pieces chicken (breast halves, whole legs), skinned
      1 large onion, chopped
      1 clove garlic, chopped
        Dash ground ginger
    ¼ teaspoon ground coriander
        Freshly ground black pepper to taste
      1 tablespoon lemon juice
    ¼ cup vinegar
      1 tablespoon oil
      3 tablespoons water
    ¼ teaspoon raw sugar
    ⅛ teaspoon cinnamon
    ½ tablespoon low-sodium beef bouillon
      1 tablespoon chopped fresh parsley

In your blender or food processor, combine all the ingredients except the chicken and parsley, and blend to a smooth paste. Place the chicken in a shallow baking dish and pierce all over with a fork. Spread with the paste. Cover and refrigerate overnight.

Preheat your oven to "Broil." When oven is ready, place chicken on broiler rack and broil for 15 minutes on each side or until chicken is brown, basting occasionally with pan-juices. When brown, remove chicken from oven, garnish with parsley, and serve.
SERVES 4

Chicken with Fried Onions

4 pieces chicken (2 breast halves, 2 whole legs), skinned
1 medium-size onion, finely chopped
Dash powdered ginger
2 large cloves garlic, peeled and chopped
2 tablespoons water
1 tablespoon unsalted margarine, softened
1 medium onion, sliced into rings
½ tablespoon plus ½ cup dry white wine
1 ½-pound eggplant, peeled and coarsely chopped
½ teaspoon cinnamon
1 tablespoon lemon juice
1 teaspoon sugar
Cayenne pepper to taste
2 potatoes, boiled, peeled, and cubed
½ red pepper, chopped
½ tablespoon low-sodium chicken bouillon
1 tablespoon nonfat plain yogurt

In your blender, purée the chopped onion, ginger, garlic, and water to a paste and set aside. Heat the margarine in a large skillet, and then fry the onion rings over a very low flame until they are wilted. Remove to paper towels and drain.

In the same skillet, brown the chicken on both sides over medium heat and remove to a platter. Add ½ tablespoon wine and the onion paste you blended before to the pan, and cook over medium heat for 5 minutes, stirring constantly.

Add the eggplant and cinnamon to the pan and stirfry for 2 minutes over low heat. Then add the lemon juice, sugar, pepper, and the remaining ½ cup of wine. Stir it all until well mixed. Add the chicken and bring the mixture to a boil. Reduce heat, add the onion rings, cover, and simmer over low heat for 30 minutes.

Now, add the potatoes and red pepper, cover, and simmer 15 minutes more. Stir in the chicken bouillon and yogurt, and the dish is done. Serve.

SERVES 4

Curried Chicken

> 1 1½-pound chicken, skinned and cut into serving
>   pieces, *or* 1½ pounds boned and skinned chicken
>   breasts
> ½ teaspoon black pepper
> 1 teaspoon garlic powder
> ½ tablespoon Dijon mustard
> ⅓ cup water
> 2 tablespoons lemon juice
> 2 tablespoons honey
> 1 tablespoon curry powder
> ½ large onion, sliced
> 2 carrots, peeled and sliced

Preheat oven to 350°.

Place the chicken pieces in a roasting pan and sprinkle half the pepper and garlic powder on top.

In a bowl, combine the mustard with 3 tablespoons water. Stir in the lemon juice, honey, and curry powder. Pour half the curry mixture over the chicken and scatter the onion and carrots around it. Pour remaining water over the vegetables (enough to cover) and bake for 30 minutes.

Then turn the chicken, and sprinkle with the remaining pepper and garlic. Pour on the remaining curry mixture. If needed, add more water to the pan. Bake 45 minutes more, or until the chicken is brown. Serve with brown rice.
SERVES 3

Chicken Kabobs

¾ pound chicken meat, cut into cubes
½ teaspoon oil or spray Pam (vegetable spray)
½ large green pepper, seeded and cut into 1-inch
    chunks
½ large onion, cut into 1-inch cubes
 8 medium-size mushroom caps, cleaned and dried
    (discard stems)
¼ teaspoon dried thyme
¼ teaspoon ground coriander
 4 bay leaves
¼ teaspoon garlic powder
¼ teaspoon mustard powder
    Freshly ground black pepper to taste
½ cup red wine
¾ tablespoon white vinegar

6–8 cherry tomatoes
  Wooden or metal skewers

In a skillet, heat the oil or spray Pam, and stir-fry green pepper, onion, and mushroom caps for about three minutes. Remove from heat and cool.

In a bowl, combine all the herbs, spices, wine, and vinegar; add stirfried vegetables and chicken, and toss. Marinate for eight hours.

Preheat broiler.

Alternately thread pieces of chicken, green pepper, tomato, onion, and mushroom cap on the skewers. Reserve the marinade.

Place skewers on broiler rack about three inches from heat and broil for 5 minutes, basting often with marinade; then turn them over and broil for another 3–5 minutes, until the kabobs look done but not dry. Serve over brown rice.
SERVES 4

Chicken Salad

1¼ cup diced cooked chicken white-meat, unsalted
  1 large apple, diced
  2 tablespoons nonfat plain yogurt
  ½ teaspoon curry powder
  ⅛ cup chopped unsalted almonds (optional)

Combine all the ingredients and serve on a bed of lettuce.
SERVES 4

Chinese Sesame-Chicken Salad

                2 cups finely shredded cooked chicken breasts
                2 tablespoons sesame seeds
                1 tablespoon Dijon mustard
                ¼ teaspoon ground ginger
                1½ teaspoons garlic powder
                1 teaspoon onion powder
                ¼ cup orange juice
                1 teaspoon low-sodium soy sauce
                2 cups finely chopped celery
                2 cups finely shredded scallions, cut into 1½-inch
                    lengths
                2 tablespoons finely chopped red pepper
                5 cups shredded crisp iceberg lettuce
                Orange slices and tomato wedges for garnish

Toast the sesame seeds until lightly browned by placing them in a small pan in a moderately hot oven or toaster oven for a few minutes; remove and let cool. (If you prefer, you can buy sesame seeds that are already roasted.)

Put the shredded chicken in a bowl and sprinkle with the mustard, ginger, garlic and onion powders, orange juice, soy sauce, and seasame seeds; toss well. Place the chicken in the refrigerator to marinate and chill, at least 15 minutes.

Meanwhile, prepare the celery, scallions, red pepper, and lettuce. When the chicken is chilled, stir in the celery, scallions, and red pepper. Arrange the lettuce on a platter and top it with the chicken salad. Garnish the platter with orange slices and tomato wedges.

SERVES 4

FISH

Broiled Fresh Salmon Steaks

You might love to know that one salmon steak cooked this way has about 300 calories.

> 2 salmon steaks
> 2 tablespoons lime juice
> 1 teaspoon unsalted margarine
> Pepper to taste
> 2 teaspoons chopped fresh tarragon, *or* ½ teaspoon dried
> ½ cup dry white wine or dry vermouth

Preheat broiler.

Place the salmon steaks in a shallow baking pan. Sprinkle with half the lime juice and dot with margarine. Season with pepper. Sprinkle with half the tarragon, and pour the wine or vermouth around but not over the salmon. Broil for 10–15 minutes, basting often during the last 5 minutes. Turn salmon, season with remaining ingredients, and broil about 5 minutes longer. Baste again when done, and remove steaks to serving dish. Pour the sauce over the steaks, and serve.
SERVES 2

Harry Alan Salmon

    2 salmon steaks
    1 teaspoon garlic powder
    2 teaspoons chopped fresh dill
      Pinch finely ground pepper
    2 tablespoons capers in their juice
    ½ lemon, thinly sliced

Preheat broiler.

Place salmon steaks on a cookie sheet. Mix garlic powder, dill, and pepper; sprinkle half the mixture and 1 tablespoon of capers and juice on top of the fish. Broil for 8 minutes. Turn the fish over, and repeat the procedure. Broil for 8–10 more minutes. Remove from heat, garnish with lemon slices, and serve.

SERVES 2

Steamed Snapper with Scallions and Ginger

    1 2-pound snapper *or* 2 snapper fillets
    1 tablespoon sesame oil
    1 teaspoon white vinegar
    2 teaspoons mustard powder
    1 tablespoon white wine
    ⅛ teaspoon ground ginger
    8 scallions, minced
    2 tablespoons low-sodium beef bouillon

In a large skillet or wok, pour water to a depth of ¾ inch. Place a steamer over the water and bring to a boil. Place fish in a glass casserole and set on the steamer. Lower the heat, cover tightly, and cook for 15 minutes.

Just before fish is done, combine and heat remaining ingredients in a small saucepan. Remove steamed fish to serving dish, and stir the remaining pan-juices into the saucepan containing the other ingredients. Pour mixture over snapper and serve.
SERVES 2

Fish Kabobs

> ½ pound sea scallops or fish fillets (swordfish or
>   halibut work well)
> 1 tablespoon lemon juice
>   Pepper to taste
>   Pinch garlic powder (optional)
> 8–10 cherry tomatoes
> 8–10 small button mushrooms, cleaned and left whole
> ½ green pepper, sliced in 1-inch pieces (optional)
> 4 small onions
>
> 2–3 wooden skewers

Preheat broiler.

If you are using fillets, cut them into 1-inch squares. Sprinkle the fillet chunks or the scallops with the lemon juice. Season with the pepper and garlic powder.

Alternately thread a piece of fish, a tomato, a mushroom, a piece of pepper, and an onion on the skewers. Place the skewers on a metal baking pan or in a glass baking dish and broil for about 5 minutes. Turn and broil for another 3 minutes. Serve over brown rice.
SERVES 2

Fish–Broccoli Rolls in Wine Sauce

> 2 fillets of sole, 3–4 ounces each
> 4 broccoli spears, with bottoms cut off
> 4 lemon slices for garnish
>
> WINE SAUCE:
> ⅓ cup water
> ¼ cup dry white wine
> ¼ cup bottled white grape juice
> 1½ tablespoon lemon juice
> ½ tablespoon plus ½ teaspoon Dijon mustard
> 1 teaspoon coarsely chopped capers, drained
> ¼ teaspoon onion powder
> ¼ teaspoon garlic powder
> 1 bay leaf
> ⅓ cup chopped scallions

Combine all the sauce ingredients except the scallions in a skillet. Cook over medium heat, stirring frequently, until thickened. Stir in the scallions. Roll each fillet around the stem of a broccoli spear; lay the rolls in the sauce, seam side down, and baste with spoonfuls of sauce. Cook, covered, over medium heat for 12 minutes. While the fish rolls cook, steam the other 2 broccoli spears until tender, just a few minutes.

When fish rolls are done, transfer to a serving dish and pour the sauce over them. Arrange the steamed broccoli spears around the fish, garnish with the lemon slices, and serve.
SERVES 2

Baked or Broiled Fish with Dill

You want simple? This is about as simple as you can get and still eat well and feel full.

> 2 fillets of fish: cod, sole, halibut, or trout
>   Pepper to taste
> 1 teaspoon chopped fresh dill, *or* ¼ teaspoon dried
> 2 tablespoons dry white wine (optional)
> 2 tablespoons fresh lemon juice
> 2 teaspoons unsalted margarine

Preheat broiler, or preheat oven to 350°, depending on chosen cooking method.

Wash the fish and dry well. Place in a glass baking pan. Sprinkle with the other ingredients, finishing off with a teaspoon of margarine on each fillet.

If you are baking, bake for 15–20 minutes. If you are broiling, do so for 8–10 minutes, watching carefully that the fish does not get too dried out (it will start to curl and brown). Serve with steamed vegetables.
SERVES 2

Seafood Salads

Four-Shrimp Salad

4 medium shrimp, cooked and cut into pieces or left
   whole
½ head red leaf or butter (Boston) lettuce
1 tablespoon chopped scallions
¼ cucumber, peeled and sliced
1 tomato, quartered
2 tablespoons Low-calorie, Low-sodium Vinaigrette
   Dressing (see page 180)

Wash and dry the lettuce, tear into bite-sized pieces, and put
in a salad bowl. Add the other ingredients, toss, and enjoy.
SERVES 1

Tuna Salad

SALAD:
½ 7-ounce can water-packed tuna, drained and flaked
1 cup bean sprouts, lightly steamed and chopped, or
   uncooked if preferred
½ cup chopped celery
¼ cup chopped green pepper
1 small scallion, chopped, *or* ¼ cup finely chopped
   white onion
1 hard-boiled egg white, chopped
1 tomato, sliced
1 large apple, peeled and grated

DRESSING:
¼ cup Low-calorie, Low-sodium Vinaigrette Dressing
     (see page 180), *or* ⅓ cup herb- or garlic-flavored
     red or white wine vinegar, plus 3 tablespoons
     water
2 teaspoons prepared mustard (regular or Dijon)

Combine all the salad ingredients in a bowl and chill well, at least 15 minutes.

Mix the dressing ingredients thoroughly and pour over the salad, tossing gently. Use as a sandwich filling or as a stuffing for a fresh tomato.
MAKES ABOUT 2 CUPS

Salade Niçoise

1 head iceberg, red leaf, or butter (Boston) lettuce
1 7-ounce can water-packed tuna
½ pound green beans, cooked
1 small onion, or ½ red onion, sliced
1 tomato, sliced
½ green pepper, seeded and cut in strips
½ red pepper, seeded and cut in strips
2 hard-boiled egg whites, sliced
2 small potatoes, boiled, skinned, and sliced
2–4 tablespoons Low-calorie, Low-sodium Vinaigrette
     Dressing (see page 180)
2 tablespoons grated Parmesan cheese (optional)

Wash lettuce and dry in a lettuce dryer or with paper towels. Tear each lettuce leaf in half; line a salad bowl with the leaves.

Drain the tuna, flake with a fork, and place around the bowl on the lettuce. Then add each of the ingredients in turn. Mix the whole salad with just enough dressing to coat but not soak the ingredients.

SERVES 2

VEGETABLES

Broccoli

Broccoli is the perfect vegetable—high in vitamin A, potassium, and calcium. And it is easy to prepare.

Start by soaking the broccoli in cold water for about 10 minutes. Drain and pat dry with a paper towel. Then remove all the leaves and cut off the bottom hard part of the stalks.

Put about 1 inch of water in a pot and bring to a boil. Add the broccoli (if you have a steamer, place the broccoli on the steamer rack in a pot). Cook for about 10 minutes, or until the broccoli is tender to your fork but not too soft.

Remove the broccoli from the pot using a fork or tongs. Sprinkle lemon juice and grated Parmesan cheese over the broccoli.

When you are on the Diet for Life, you have several additional options. You can add margarine (1 tablespoon should be enough for most portions) and 1 teaspoon lemon juice. Also try margarine and ¼ teaspoon dried dill; margarine and ¼ teaspoon dried basil; or margarine with any other spices or herbs that you like, such as oregano, curry, rosemary, etc.

Steamed Vegetable Plate

> ANY COMBINATION OF THE FOLLOWING
> VEGETABLES:
>   Broccoli
>   Potatoes
>   Zucchini
>   Tomatoes
>   Carrots
>   Squash
>   Fresh spinach leaves, cleaned well
> 2–4 tablespoons chopped fresh parsley
>   1 tablespoon grated Parmesan cheese

Wash the chosen vegetables well, then peel and/or slice into bite-sized pieces.

Place the vegetables in 1 inch of water in a pot, on a steamer if you have one, and put on your stove over a low flame. Cook until the vegetables can be pricked by a fork but are not too soft. (A hint: After so many years of steaming vegetables, I have developed a method to my madness. Since some vegetables get steamed faster than others, I usually put the carrots, potatoes, and broccoli in first. Then, after 3–4 minutes, I add the zucchini, spinach, and squash. That way they all get done to a similar consistency, with none of them being too well done. However, if you are not as picky as I am, just put them all in at once. They will still be as nutritious and as delicious.)

When the vegetables are done, remove from the pot and place in a serving dish. Sprinkle with chopped parsley or Parmesan cheese (never salt!). If you are on the Diet for Life, you can add 1 tablespoon margarine.

Broiled Tomato Halves with Garlic

>   2 large ripe tomatoes
>   1 teaspooon melted unsalted margarine
>   1 clove garlic, minced
>   ¼ teaspoon summer savory
>   ¼ teaspoon dried thyme
>   ¾ cup fresh coarsely grated Parmesan cheese
>   1 small yellow or green squash, sliced and steamed
>   Parsley sprigs

Preheat broiler.

Cut the tomatoes in half vertically and arrange on a baking sheet, cut side up. Mix the melted margarine with the garlic and herbs, and spread mixture onto cut surfaces of tomatoes. Sprinkle thickly with cheese.

Place under the broiler and cook until the cheese is melted and golden brown, 10–12 minutes. I like the tomato garnished with steamed slices of yellow squash and parsley sprigs. It's pretty and adds a healthy touch.
SERVES 3

Vegetable Salad

*ANY COMBINATION OF THE FOLLOWING
VEGETABLES:*
　　Zucchini
　　Green peppers
　　Broccoli
　　Mushrooms
　　Carrots
　　Tomatoes
1 head Boston (butter) or red leaf lettuce
¼ cup chopped scallions
1 tablespoon chopped fresh parsley
2 tablespoons low-cal, low-sodium dressing of your
　　choice

Clean as many of the vegtables as you want, and cut them into small pieces.

Wash and dry the lettuce, tear into bite-sized pieces, and put in a salad bowl. Add the scallions, parsley, and prepared vegetables. Toss with the dressing and serve.
SERVES 2–4

Italian Vegetable Salad

                4 tomatoes, quartered
                ½ cucumber, peeled and sliced
                1 small green pepper, sliced
                ¼ pound button mushrooms, sliced
                2 tablespoons wine vinegar
                1 teaspoon olive oil
                    Freshly ground black pepper to taste
                1 tablespoon chopped fresh parsley
                1 tablespoon lemon juice
                1 hard-boiled egg white, sliced
                ½ head lettuce

Put the tomatoes, cucumber, green pepper, and mushrooms in a salad bowl and toss with the vinegar, oil, and black pepper. Refrigerate for 15–30 minutes. Take from refrigerator, add the parsley, and mix. Sprinkle the lemon juice over the top, garnish with the egg white slices and serve over lettuce.
SERVES 2–4, depending on how much lettuce you use.

Spinach–Mushroom Salad

                ½ pound fresh spinach leaves, well washed
                ¼ pound button mushrooms, sliced
                2 tablespoons chopped scallions
                ¼ teaspoon low-sodium soy sauce
                2 tablespoons Low-calorie, Low-sodium Vinaigrette
                    Dressing (see page 180)
                1 hard-boiled egg white, sliced

Make sure you wash the spinach leaves well—they tend to be very dirty. (I soak mine in cold water for about five minutes, then rinse under running water.) Dry the leaves in paper towels or in a lettuce dryer. Put them in a salad bowl and add the mushrooms and scallions.

Add the soy sauce to the vinaigrette. Sprinkle over the salad and toss well. Garnish with the egg white slices and serve.
SERVES 1–2

Garden Green Salad

> ½ head lettuce
> 2 tablespoons chopped scallions
> 1 tablespoon chopped fresh parsley
> 2 tablespoons chopped celery (optional)
> ½ cucumber, peeled and sliced (optional)
> ½ green pepper, sliced (optional)
> ½ zucchini, sliced (optional)
> 2 tablespoons Low-calorie, Low-sodium Vinaigrette
> Dressing (see page 242)

Wash the lettuce well, then dry in a lettuce dryer or on paper towels. (You can keep the lettuce refrigerated, wrapped in paper towels, until you are ready to make your salad.)

Tear the lettuce leaves (in salad making, there are two schools of lettuce followers—one says you should cut the lettuce with a knife, the other swears you should tear the lettuce with your hands. I prefer tearing—you do it any way you like!) and put them in a salad bowl. Add the rest of the ingredients you have chosen and toss. Now add the dressing (1 or 2 tablespoons should be enough, but you can add a drop more if you like), toss again, and serve.
SERVES 1–2

Sliced Tomato Salad

This is as easy as it sounds. First, take one or two tomatoes and slice them thinly. Next, if you like lettuce, you can add 3 or 4 leaves of red leaf or butter lettuce; also optional are chopped scallions. But be careful or this can turn into a "green salad." Add a little Low-calorie, Low-sodium vinaigrette (see page 180), and a pinch of black pepper. That's it! If you think this sounds like a boring lunch, try it. You'll find that tomatoes are delicious all by themselves.

Eggs

Scrambled Egg White

> 1 egg white
>   Dab unsalted margarine

Melt the margarine in a small frying pan (use just enough to coat pan so egg doesn't stick). Add the egg white and cook over low flame until the white starts to set. Flip it over and cook until done (just like a fried egg, but without the yolk). Serve on dry wheat toast, with tomato slices

Mini Omelette

> 2 egg whites
> 1 egg yolk
>   Dab unsalted margarine

In a small mixing bowl, hand beat the egg whites and yolk. Then, in a small frying pan over medium heat, melt the margarine and pour in the egg mixture. You can scramble the eggs or make an omelette by merely turning it over once.

If you like your eggs seasoned, you can serve this omelette with Salsa (see page 184) on the side. If you really must, you can add a pinch of salt and pepper for added seasoning. The point here is to minimize the fat content of the egg but still get the protein.

Eggs Florentine

> ½ pound fresh leaf spinach, *or* 1 box frozen leaf
>   spinach, thawed
> ¼ teaspoon raw sugar
>   Pepper to taste
> 2 tablespoons unsalted margarine
> 4 eggs
> 2 tablespoons grated Parmesan cheese
> ½ cup nonfat plain yogurt

Steam the spinach; drain, pressing well, and season with the sugar and pepper. Place in a heated gratin dish, dot with margarine, and make four holes in the spinach. Poach the eggs, and lay one in each of the hollowed "nests."

Preheat broiler.

In a small pan, mix half the cheese with the yogurt and cook, stirring, for 2 minutes over medium heat. Spoon the yogurt mixture over the eggs and spinach. Sprinkle the remaining cheese on top. Put under the broiler to melt the cheese, just 30 seconds to 1 minute, and serve immediately.

SERVES 4

EXTRAS

Banana Bread

This bread is delicious as a dessert, for breakfast, or to carry around with you for a bag lunch or a snack during the day.

½ cup unsalted margarine, softened
¾ cup brown sugar
1 egg
1 cup unsifted whole wheat flour
½ cup unsifted unbleached white flour
1 teaspooon baking soda
¼ teaspoons cinnamon
3 ripe bananas, mashed
¼ cup nonfat plain yogurt
1 cup chopped walnuts (optional)

Preheat oven to 350°

In the blender or food processor, cream the margarine and sugar until smooth and light brown in color, then blend in the egg.

In a bowl, sift together the flours, baking soda, and cinnamon. In another bowl, mix by hand (or in the food processor) the bananas and yogurt. Then to the margarine mixture alternately add portions of the banana mixture and the flours, mixing thoroughly after each addition. Stir in walnuts, if using.

Grease a 9"- × -5" loaf pan. Pour the mixture into the pan and bake for 45 minutes to an hour. (You can test the bread's readiness by pricking it with a knife—if it comes out clean, the bread is ready. If not, return it to the oven for another 10 minutes.)

After you remove the bread from the oven, let it stand for about 15 minutes to cool. Then remove it from the pan and let it stand for about an hour so it won't crumble when you try to cut it.

MAKES 1 LOAF

Tomato Dressing for Salad

    1 cup tomato juice
    1 clove garlic, peeled and pressed
    1 tablespoon chopped fresh parsley
    1 tablespoon chopped fresh chives
    ½ teaspoon Dijon mustard
       Freshly ground black pepper to taste
       Pinch raw sugar

Mix all the ingredients together in a small bowl with a wire whisk, or in your food processor. Put in your refrigerator in a covered glass jar until ready to use (the dressing tastes better after it has been sitting for a while). For a salad for two people, 1 tablespoon of the dressing is enough. Remember, you don't want the lettuce drenched with the dressing—just coated with it.

MAKES 1 CUP

THE BIKINI DIET

Let's get it straight right up front—I do not believe in crash diets. Basically, they are dangerous, and they don't work because people tend to go back to their old habits and gain back the weight they lost. Thus most crash diets are temporary, and unsuccessful.

However, the Bikini Diet, because it is based on the Diet Principles and derived from the 30-Day Diet to Lose, is not dangerous if followed exactly as prescribed and *only for seven days*, after which you go immediately to the 30-Day Diet to Lose. (Make yourself a note to try to go on the diet between menstrual cycles so you are not losing blood while you are on it.)

The Bikini Diet is an emergency diet. It is designed only for those times in your life when you must take off 5–10 pounds in a short period of time. I have used this diet when I gained an extra 5 pounds and needed to take them off for a photo session, and in order to make the first spring appearance in a movie. But I have never gone on this diet more than *twice a year!*

The diet itself will be familiar to those of you who have tried or read the 30-Day Diet to Lose. The principles are basically the same, as are the foods (and therefore the recipes). It is only the amounts which are different.

The wonderful thing about this diet, other than the fact that it is immediately effective, is that it is not a starvation diet—it's very low-calorie and low-bulk, while at the same time still high in nutrients. As with the other diets, it is important to eat the foods exactly as listed—don't ever try to eat less! And if you find that you don't feel well while on this diet, stop and see your doctor.

THE PRINCIPLES

1. As I advised with the 30-Day Diet to Lose, see your doctor before starting this diet. Anyone who is not in good physical condition as defined by a doctor should not attempt any diet. When your doctor gives you the go-ahead, you can start.

2. Follow the diet to a "T." Don't deviate from the prescribed menu for this seven-day period. This is not the time to experiment, let alone to cheat. I am assuming that you are definitely dedicated and absolutely determined to lose that extra weight in a hurry, and that you need to do so fast and safely (otherwise you should be on the 30-Day Diet to Lose). So follow the menu; besides, you'll find it easier to eat exactly what the diet calls for.

3. Never eat after eight o'clock in the evening. Start your dinner earlier so your body has the time to digest the meal before you go to bed.

4. I don't believe in prescribing the weight of the foods you should eat. I have never weighed food in my life—it is a chore I don't have the time or the inclination for. I merely measure by the slice—if your slice is bigger than mine, that's fine. If your slice is closer to half a chicken, think again before you take a bite, and then cut.

5. Eat wheat toast with fiber in it (you can find it in any supermarket). Take the trouble to find it and to eat it—your body needs the fiber and this is a good way to get it. Don't skip the bread and think you are doing yourself a favor.

6. As I explained in the 30-Day Diet to Lose, I don't think coffee is good for you, so I don't drink it. Tea is my drink—it flushes out the system and if you drink it light the intake of caffeine is minimal.

7. Ask your doctor about calcium supplements. Even the government has recently agreed that women need calcium in large amounts (at least 1200 mgs. a day, as advised by the FDA), and you can't get it all from drinking milk or eating cheese. Since I believe that the fat in dairy foods is bad for your system and your looks, I consume very few dairy products and none at all during the Bikini Diet. So especially during this week, be sure to take your calcium supplements.

8. No canned food at all during this diet, except for tuna which should be water packed. Every other ingredient should be fresh.

9. For salads, use only low-cal dressings. No more cream dressings—not even the so-called "low-cal cream" dressings. Stick to the other low-cal and diet dressings. You'll get less fat and less sodium, neither of which your body needs.

10. No alcohol for the seven days—not even beer. Its extra calories are unnecessary. Remember, you are losing extra weight and also flushing out your system. What you don't need is any alcohol to get in the way. There is plenty of time for that during the Diet for Life, where my recipes use wines and liquors as wonderful taste additives.

11. Try to eat at home as much as possible during the seven days. This will minimize any temptations and will also put the control of what you put in your body firmly in your hands. But if you find yourself in a restaurant, don't panic. Relax and simply order the food prescribed in the diet. You'll find that any restaurant can give you a salad without dressing, plain broiled chicken or fish, etc. It's usually no problem and no one minds, so don't hesitate to ask for what you want.

12. If you are addicted to diet sodas, this is a good time to wean yourself from them. Iced tea works better to flush out your system, and diet sodas add nothing to a diet except a lot of gas. Later, when you are on the Diet for Life, you can go back to occasional sodas (after all, remember, I don't believe in a life of total denial—just in a smarter allocation of our resources!).

13. Don't be afraid to season your foods. Herbs add taste to any food without adding additional calories.

THE DIET

Important: Look up Basic Beverage Rule on page 87 and follow it to the letter!

BREAKFAST	**LUNCH**	**DINNER**
DAY 1		
Scrambled Egg White (p. 112)	Salad made with any vegetables except tomatoes	Steamed Vegetable Plate (p. 107)
1 slice wheat toast, dry	1 slice turkey (optional)	Beverage
Beverage	Beverage	
DAY 2		
1 glass prune juice	Salad made with lettuce, tomato, ⅓ cup tuna (low-cal dressing, optional)	1 cup low-sodium chicken broth
1 slice wheat toast, dry		Steamed celery
Beverage		1 slice chicken (white meat)
	Beverage	Beverage

BREAKFAST	LUNCH	DINNER
DAY 3		
1 sliced whole tomato on dry wheat toast (low-cal Italian dressing, optional) Beverage	½ cup Chicken Salad (p. 97) 2 melba toasts Beverage	½ cup any Steamed Vegetables (p. 107) Beverage
DAY 4		
Scrambled Egg White (p. 112) 1 slice wheat toast, dry Beverage	1 cup any steamed or raw vegetables Beverage	broiled fish 2 melba toasts 1 cup steamed broccoli or zucchini Beverage
DAY 5		
1 glass prune juice 1 slice wheat toast, dry Beverage	Salad made with ½ cup shrimp, and sliced mushrooms, tomatoes, lettuce (low-cal dressing, optional) Beverage	1½ cups any Steamed Vegetables (p. 107) Beverage
DAY 6		
½ cup cut melon or strawberries 1 slice wheat toast, dry Beverage	1 cup diced chicken and tomato 1 melba toast Beverage	broiled fish ½ sliced tomato, low-cal dressing Beverage
DAY 7		
½ tomato, sliced or 1 slice melon 1 slice wheat toast, dry Beverage	1 cup Tuna or Chicken Salad (pp. 97, 104) Beverage	broiled chicken 1 cup steamed broccoli or cauliflower 2 melba toasts Beverage

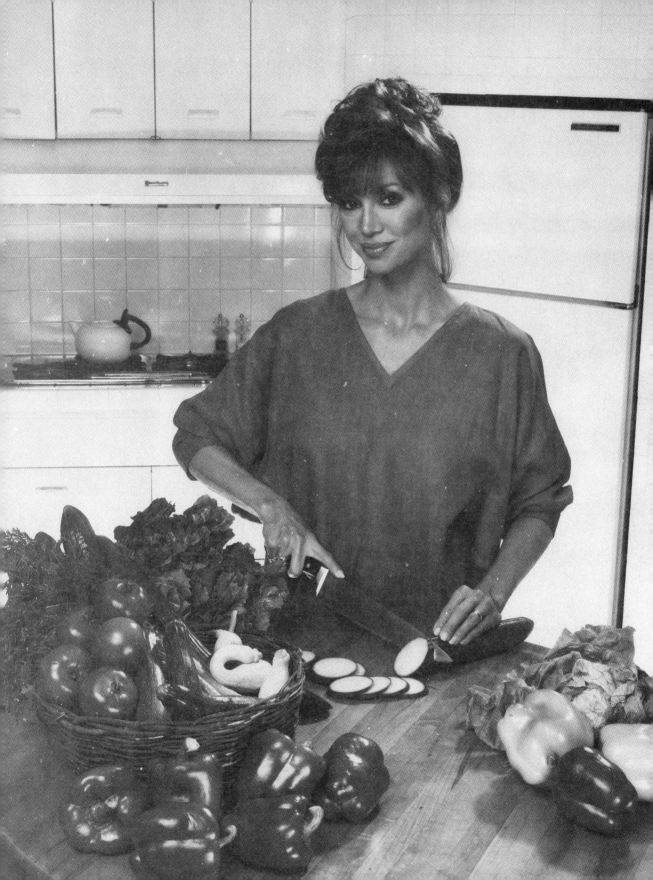

CHAPTER 4

THE DIET FOR LIFE

The Diet for Life is a philosophy of eating that will carry you through the rest of your life. Basically everything in this book has been leading up to this diet; part of the diet is in the Diet Principles, part in the chapter on the philosophy of nutrition, and part in the rules for the 30-Day Diet to Lose on how to eat in a healthier way.

The diet is a "style of eating" that lets you keep and control your healthy and comfortable weight forever. Should you cheat a little and gain some unwanted weight, you can easily go right on the 30-Day Diet to Lose and then back again when you've lost the desired weight.

A balanced diet composed of these dishes will contain all the nutrients your body needs. The recipes are made up of the "Perfect" and the "Maybe/Sometimes" foods. However, when you find that you want a chocolate eclair or a hot dog, go ahead and eat one. Don't feel guilty; don't reproach yourself. If you are going to eat something that is "special" to you, at least enjoy it! Just remember to compensate as soon as you can. For example, if you eat a hot dog for lunch on a given day, try to stick to a vegetable dish and/or a salad for dinner. Or if you gorge on a dessert at dinner, try to eat a leaner, no-sugar breakfast and lunch the next day, and make the time for some sort of exercise. You see how it works.

Remember, you are now in total control of what you put into your body. You know what is in the foods you eat (and in those you don't want to pass your lips too often); you know the guidelines for eating well-balanced and nutritious meals; you understand the value and importance of the diet princi-ples, and you know too that they apply to eating for life. Thus, now is the time to trust your own newly developed and ex-panded judgments as to what you should eat, when you should eat, and how much you should eat.

As you know by now, I refuse to count calories or weigh food. I firmly believe (and I have long practiced) that using my knowledge about foods and "dieting" is enough. I have re-sisted the concept of laying everything out in terms of ounces and calories because you can't carry this book around with you for the rest of your lives. What I have done is give you a basic understanding of your nutritional requirements, and guidelines on how to meet them without overeating. I know how much is too much—and so will you.

With this new knowledge and some common sense you can eat happily and healthfully for the rest of your life. But re-member—be honest! If you try to fool yourself even a little bit, those pounds will creep back on sooner than you can imagine!

Here too, as in the 30-Day Diet to Lose, moderation, variety and balance are the key ingredients. The Diet for Life recipes are balanced for nutrients and for variety of foods. You are in charge of the "moderation" part; as long as you eat all but the very terrible foods in moderation (this doesn't mean twice a day—not even twice a week!) and learn how to compensate every now and then, you'll be healthy and happy (I hope) and thin.

In this chapter you will find all the recipes that are part of the Diet for Life. They are catalogued simply, according to food group, and are made of all the delicious and nutritious foods you can eat forever. You should note that while you should not eat these foods while you are on the 30-Day Diet to Lose, you can however add the recipes from that diet to this group. Thus any dish that is on the 30-Day Diet to Lose can be made while you are on the Diet for Life maintenance program. Simply make some intelligent additions to the "diet" meal. I should also mention that you can add any other recipes you collect from other books and from your friends and relatives as long as they fit into your new knowledge about good nutrition and healthy eating.

In order to give you an idea of a typical week of Diet for Life menus, I have included a sample "7-Day Diet for Life." If you wish, you can follow it the first week after you have completed the 30-Day Diet to Lose, but it is intended more as an example of what and how you can expect to eat for the rest of your life. As you'll quickly find out, there's plenty to choose from— there's not a chance you'll feel the least bit deprived!

So go to it—enjoy the meals, knowing full well that the foods you are eating are as healthy (and as delicious) as they can be.

SAMPLE MENU—THE DIET FOR LIFE

Important: Don't forget to follow the Basic Beverage Rule outlined on page 87.

BREAKFAST	LUNCH	DINNER
DAY 1		
Banana Yogurt Breakfast (p. 217)	Tuna Salad with Dressing (p. 104)	Herb Chicken (p. 140)
1 or 2 slices wheat toast, dry	Unsalted crackers	Broccoli
1 glass nonfat milk	Beverage	Sautéed Cherry Tomatoes (p. 205)
Hot tea (sugar OK for the first cup; then use sweetener)		Small green salad
		Beverage
DAY 2		
1 bowl cereal (like Bran Flakes or Cheerios)	Sliced chicken plate (with mustard, if you like)	Grilled Swordfish (p. 154)
½ small melon filled with strawberries, raspberries, blueberries, etc.	Sliced Tomato Salad (p. 112)	Curried Spinach Rice (p. 191)
1 glass nonfat milk	1 slice bread (or you can have a sliced chicken sandwich)	Broccoli
Hot tea		1 slice bread (skip if you had 2 at lunch)
	Beverage	Beverage
DAY 3		
Good-for-You French Toast (p. 217)	Cold salmon plate or salmon salad sandwich	Chicken or Turkey Salad with No-Guilt Dressing (p. 180)
½ melon	Sliced cucumbers/ tomatoes	1 Honey Apple (p. 211)
1 glass nonfat milk	Beverage	Beverage
Hot tea		

BREAKFAST	LUNCH	DINNER
DAY 4		
Omelette (1 egg; if you want 2, only use the white of the second egg—see p. 112) with mushrooms, peppers, tomatoes, onions 1 slice wheat toast 1 glass nonfat milk Hot tea	Italian Vegetable Salad (p. 110) Unsalted crackers Beverage	Veal Scallops in Tomato Sauce (p. 175) Boiled or baked potato Steamed spinach with lemon Sliced Tomato Salad (p. 112) (lettuce OK) 1 fresh orange, sliced Beverage
DAY 5		
Berry Bran Muffin (p. 207) ½ small melon 1 glass nonfat milk Hot tea	Tomato stuffed with Tuna Salad (p. 104) or Chicken Salad (p. 97) Unsalted crackers Beverage	Steamed Vegetable Plate (p. 107) with potato or pasta Breadsticks 1 sliced peach or Pears in Rum (p. 214) Beverage
DAY 6		
Fruit salad 1 Popover (p. 209) or 1 slice wheat toast 1 glass nonfat milk Hot tea	Caesar or Shrimp Salad (p. 104) Unsalted crackers Beverage	Veal Picatta (p. 174) Spaghetti with Asparagus (p. 190) Garden Green Salad (p. 111) Breadsticks Beverage
DAY 7		
1 bagel, lox, a tiny bit of cream cheese Sliced tomato and onion 1 glass ice water Hot tea	Garden Green Salad (p. 111) with sliced turkey Vegetables Beverage	Marinated Bass Teriyaki (p. 170) Orange-Flavored Rice (p. 192) Broccoli Banana–Berry Dessert (p. 212) Beverage

SOUPS

Bean Soup

1 15-ounce can red kidney beans
1 15-ounce can pinto beans
1 15-ounce can wax beans
1 tablespoon olive oil
1 large onion, chopped
1 teaspoon celery powder
1 cup sliced carrots
4–6 cups low-sodium chicken broth
1 16-ounce can Italian plum tomatoes, drained and
    chopped
1 bay leaf
1 teaspoon dried basil
½ teaspoon dried rosemary
½ teaspoon dried oregano
    Freshly ground black pepper to taste
½ cup vermouth

Drain all the beans in a large colander.

In a large pot over medium heat, heat the oil, and add the onion and celery powder. Sauté until the onions are soft but not brown. Now add the carrots and cook another 5 minutes. Add the drained beans, 4 cups of the chicken broth, the tomatoes, the herbs, and the pepper, and cook, uncovered, for 30 minutes over a low flame. At this point, check the soup —if the liquid has boiled down too much and the soup is getting too thick for your taste, add another 1 or 2 cups chicken broth. Add the vermouth, and continue cooking for another 15 minutes.

That's it—except for remembering to remove the bay leaf when the soup is done.
SERVES 6–8

Note: I often freeze what's left of the soup. When I defrost it, I cream it in the food processor and have Cream of Bean Soup. It's terrific!

Iced Cucumber Soup

> 1 small onion, finely chopped
> 1 tablespoon safflower oil
> 1 large cucumber, peeled and sliced
> 4 medium potatoes, sliced
> 3 cups chicken stock
>   Pinch white pepper
> 2 tablespoons nonfat plain yogurt
> 2 tablespoons chopped mint and/or scallions

In a large saucepan over medium heat, sauté the onion in the oil, then add the cucumber and potatoes. Reduce heat and cook very gently for 10 minutes, stirring from time to time; avoid browning. Add the stock and pepper and bring to a boil. Cover, lower heat, and simmer gently for 20 minutes.

Blend the soup in a food processor or blender, and pour into a bowl to cool. When it is cold, you may want to adjust the seasonings to taste. (Just be gentle with your craving for salt —this soup really doesn't need it.) Refrigerate until ready to serve.

Just before serving, stir in the yogurt and garnish with chopped mint and/or scallions. Serve chilled.
SERVES 6

Note: You can keep this in the refrigerator for up to 2 days.

Spinach Soup

1 small onion, chopped
1 tablespoon unsalted margarine
1 tablespoon flour
1 10-ounce package finely chopped frozen spinach,
    defrosted
2 cups chicken stock
½ cup nonfat plain yogurt

In a large saucepan over medium heat, sauté the onion in the margarine. Stir in the flour and cook for 1 minute. Now stir in the spinach and cook over low heat for 3 minutes, stirring. Add the stock and bring to a boil, then cover, lower heat, and simmer gently for 10 minutes.

Just before serving, remove from the heat and stir in the yogurt.
SERVES 2–4

Note: You can refrigerate this for up to 2 days.

Fresh Tomato Soup

I love this soup—it is healthy, low in calories, and simply delicious.

4 ripe tomatoes, roughly chopped
1 small onion, chopped
1 tablespoon vegetable oil
¼ cup orange juice
3 cups chicken stock
2 cloves garlic, each cut in half
½ teaspoon whole cloves

Bouquet garni (available in ready-made packages in
supermarket spice sections)
4 lemon slices
1 tablespoon chopped fresh dill, *or* ¼ teaspoon dried

In a large pot over medium heat, sauté the tomatoes and onion
in the oil for about 5 minutes. Add the orange juice, stock,
garlic, cloves, and *bouquet garni* to the tomato mixture. Bring
to a boil; then cover, lower heat, and simmer gently for 25
minutes. Remove the cloves and *bouquet garni*. Blend the soup
in your food processor. When you are ready to serve, reheat,
add the lemon slices, sprinkle with dill, and pour into individual soup bowls.

If you like, you can chill the soup in your refrigerator and
serve it cold.
SERVES 8

Quick Tomato Soup

½ cup finely chopped onion
1 tablespoon unsalted margarine
1 16-ounce can low-sodium tomatoes
2 tablespoons white wine
1 tablespoon chopped fresh dill, *or* ¼ teaspoon dried
1 tablespoon chopped fresh basil, *or* ¼ teaspoon dried
1 tablespoon chopped fresh parsley
2 tablespoons nonfat plain yogurt

Sauté onion in margarine until tender. Add tomatoes, wine,
dill, basil, and parsley. Simmer 20 minutes. Pour into serving
dishes and top with yogurt.
SERVES 2

Vegetable Minestrone Soup

This is, without doubt, the best minestrone soup you have ever tasted! And it doesn't have an ounce of meat in it.

> ¼ cup olive oil or unsalted margarine
> 2 onions, thinly sliced
> 2 cups sliced carrots
> 2 cups peeled and diced potatoes
> 3 florets broccoli, cut up
> 4 green zucchini, sliced
> 2 cups cut-up green beans, *or* 1 10-ounce package
>   frozen green beans
> 6 cups low-sodium chicken broth
> 1 16-ounce can Italian plum tomatoes, drained and
>   cut up
> ¼ teaspoon celery powder
> 1 10-ounce package frozen spinach, unthawed
> 1 15-ounce can pinto beans, drained
> 1 15-ounce can red kidney beans, drained
> 1 cup uncooked macaroni, any size
> ⅓ cup grated Parmesan cheese, optional

Heat the oil or margarine in a very large pot over medium heat. The cooking method is easy to remember—add each of the vegetables in turn and cook each for 3–4 minutes. Start with the onions, and cook until soft. Now add the carrots and cook; then add the potatoes, broccoli, zucchini, and green beans in turn. Next, add the chicken broth, tomatoes, and celery powder, and let the whole concoction cook over a low flame for an hour.

Now add the spinach, still frozen, and cook for 10 minutes. Add the beans and macaroni and cook for another 10 minutes. If you find the soup getting too thick, just add a cup of water.

Serve hot, topped with grated Parmesan cheese.
SERVES 8–10

Note: When I make this, I put about 4 cups of the soup in a covered plastic container and refrigerate it. Then I put the rest in freezer containers in my freezer. Sometimes weeks later, I defrost the soup and either eat it just the way it is or blend it in the food processor for a fabulous "cream of vegetable" soup.

Yogurt Soup

My friend Annie has this for breakfast almost every day. It takes all kinds . . .

> 3 medium cucumbers
> 1 pint nonfat plain yogurt
> 1 clove garlic, pressed
> 1 tablespoon vinegar
> 1 teaspoon chopped fresh dill, *or* ½ teaspoon dried
> 3 tablespoons water
> 1 tablespoon chopped fresh mint leaves, *or* ½ teaspoon
>   dried mint

Peel the cucumbers, quarter lengthwise, and slice. Place in a large bowl. Now put the yogurt, garlic, vinegar, dill, and water in your blender or food processor and blend. Pour mixture over the cucumbers and let sit for 5 minutes; then pour into soup bowls and garnish with mint. Serve.
SERVES 6

CHICKEN AND TURKEY

Chicken Breasts with Apples

The apple and lemon juice give the chicken an added tartness that I like.

> 2 whole chicken breasts, halved, boned, skinned, and
>   pounded flat (your butcher can do this for you)
> 1 medium apple, peeled and cored
> 2 tablespoons lemon juice
> 2 tablespoons unsalted margarine
> 1 onion, finely chopped
> 2 cloves garlic, peeled and pressed
> ¼ cup plain bread crumbs
> ¼ teaspoon dried rosemary, crushed
> 1 tablespoon chopped fresh basil, *or* ½ teaspoon dried
> 3 tablespoons flour
> ½ cup unsweetened apple juice
> 2 tablespoons brandy

Chop the apple in the food processor, or grate it with a grater, and put on a dish. Add the lemon juice (this will prevent the apple from turning brown), and set aside.

In a skillet over medium heat, melt half the margarine and sauté the onion and garlic until soft but not brown. Now add the apple, bread crumbs, rosemary, and basil. Cook for about 3 minutes.

Coat the chicken with flour. Melt remaining margarine in another skillet, add the chicken, and brown on both sides. Cook for about 20 minutes. Now add the apple mixture, apple juice, and brandy. Cover and simmer for another 10 minutes.

When done, put on a serving platter and serve with brown rice. A side dish of broccoli or carrots is terrific with this favorite.
SERVES 4

Chicken Breasts with Honey

   2 chicken breasts, skinned and boned
½ cup honey
¼ cup lime juice
¼ cup salad oil
   1 medium onion, diced
   1 tablespoon unsalted margarine
    Freshly ground black pepper to taste

In a medium bowl, mix the honey, lime, and oil until well blended. Add the onion and the chicken, turning the breasts to coat them thoroughly. Marinate for 30 minutes.

Preheat the broiler.

Grease a glass baking dish with the margarine. Remove the chicken from the marinade, reserving the marinade, and place chicken in the baking dish. Sprinkle the chicken with pepper. Place dish in the preheated broiler and broil until the chicken is browned, basting with the marinade and turning frequently. (This takes 15–25 minutes, but I hesitate to give you an exact time because I have found from experience that broilers are unpredictable. To be safe, I always watch the chicken to make sure it doesn't burn.)

That's it. This is delicious with a baked potato and carrots.
SERVES 2

Chicken Cacciatore

>   1 1½ pound frying chicken, skinned and cut into
>   serving pieces
>   Freshly ground black pepper to taste
>   1–2 tablespoons unsalted margarine
>   ½ pound fresh mushrooms, sliced
>   1 small onion, minced
>   1 cup plus 1 tablespoon low-sodium chicken
>   bouillon
>   ¼ cup white wine or dry vermouth
>   1 teaspoon cornstarch
>   1 tablespoon cognac
>   1 cup canned Italian plum tomatoes, drained
>   1 package frozen peas, cooked (optional)
>   2 tablespoons chopped fresh parsley
>   2 tablespoons chopped fresh basil

Wash the chicken and season with pepper. In a large skillet over high heat, melt the margarine and brown the chicken on all sides for about 20 minutes. Remove from heat and set aside in a warm place.

Add the mushrooms and onion to the skillet with one tablespoon each of the bouillon and wine, and sauté for 5 minutes until the onions are translucent, stirring and scraping the pan to loosen any browned particles. Reduce heat to low, add the cornstarch, and stir constantly for two more minutes.

Add the remaining chicken bouillon, wine, cognac, and tomatoes, and bring to a boil; then cover and simmer over low heat for 10 minutes. Add the browned chicken pieces to the wine mixture, cover, and simmer over low heat for 30 minutes or until the chicken is tender. Transfer the chicken pieces to a platter, sprinkle with the cooked peas, if using, and keep warm in your oven at 250°. Leave the sauce in the skillet.

When you are ready to serve, reduce the sauce over high heat for about five minutes. Remove from heat and add half of the parsley and basil. Pour the sauce over the chicken pieces and garnish with the remaining parsley and basil. Serve hot with rice or plain pasta.
SERVES 2–4

Chicken Provençal

2 whole chicken breasts, halved and skinned
2 tablespoons unsalted margarine
Freshly ground pepper to taste
½ cup finely chopped onion
1 large ripe tomato, coarsely chopped, *or* 8 cherry tomatoes, cut in half
½ cup canned tomato sauce
2 cloves garlic, minced
¾–1¼ cups dry white wine (may need more if it evaporates)
½ cup low-sodium chicken broth
2 small zucchini sliced into ¼-inch thick "coins"
½ pound mushrooms, sliced ½-inch thick
½ tablespoon chopped fresh chives
½ tablespoon chopped fresh parsley
½ teaspoon dried tarragon

In a large skillet or paella pan, melt half the margarine over medium heat. Sprinkle pepper on the chicken and fry two of the breasts till both sides are browned, about fifteen minutes. Remove to a platter. In the same skillet, melt the remaining margarine and brown the other two breasts in the same manner. Remove to the platter.

Add the onion, tomato, tomato sauce, and garlic to the skillet, and cook over low heat for five minutes, stirring occasionally. Return the chicken to the skillet, add ¾ cup wine and chicken broth, cover, and simmer for fifteen minutes.

Add the zucchini, mushrooms, and herbs, cover, and simmer for another 10–15 minutes. Serve over brown rice.
SERVES 4

Chicken with Red Wine

4–6 pieces of chicken, skinned
   Freshly ground black pepper to taste
1 teaspoon unsalted margarine
1 teaspoon olive oil
2 shallots, *or* 1 small white onion, coarsely chopped
1 carrot, thinly sliced
2 tablespoons cognac
2 tomatoes, peeled, seeded, and chopped, *or* 1 16-
   ounce can Italian plum tomatoes, drained and
   sliced
   Bouquet garni, or 1 tablespoon Fines Herbes (both
   available from Spice Islands)
¼ cup red wine, plus some extra wine or chicken
   stock if necessary

Season the chicken with pepper. Heat margarine and oil in a heavy casserole over medium heat, add shallots and carrot, and cook, stirring constantly, until they are soft. Then add the chicken pieces and brown on all sides.

Pour the cognac over the chicken and carefully light with a match. Now add the tomatoes, *bouquet garni* or herb mixture, and red wine. Cover the pan and let the chicken simmer over low heat until tender, about 15–20 minutes. Add more wine or some chicken stock if the sauce reduces too quickly while cooking. Serve with brown rice and a vegetable.
SERVES 2

Chicken Vera Cruz

> 4–6 pieces of chicken, skinned
> 2 tablespoons unsalted margarine
> 1 tablespoon oil
> ½ teaspoon freshly ground black pepper
> ⅓ cup brandy
> 4 cloves garlic, pressed
> 2 tablespoons chopped yellow chilis
> 2 6-ounce cans unsweetened frozen orange juice, undiluted
> ½ cup slivered almonds
> 1 orange, sliced

Wash and dry the chicken, and season with the pepper. Melt the margarine and oil in a large skillet over medium heat, and sauté the chicken in it until golden brown on all sides. Pour the brandy over the chicken and carefully set it aflame with a match. When the flames die down, add the garlic and chilis.

Blend in the undiluted orange juice and simmer for about 25 minutes, turning often to coat the chicken.

When the chicken is tender, remove it to a serving platter and pour the sauce over it. Cover with the chopped nuts and garnish with the orange slices.
SERVES 2–3

Herb Chicken

1 3½-pound chicken, cut in pieces and skinned
1 teaspoon dried marjoram
1 teaspoon dried thyme
1 tablespoon chopped fresh parsley
   Freshly ground black pepper
2 tablespoons unsalted margarine

Preheat oven to 400°.

Wash and dry the chicken. Place in a greased low baking dish and rub with marjoram and thyme. Let stand for one hour, then sprinkle with parsley and pepper and dot with margarine.

Bake in the oven for 40 minutes. Serve.
SERVES 2–4

Jade Empress Chicken

1 whole boneless chicken breast, skinned and cut
    in 1-inch cubes
¼ cup dry sherry
¼–½ tablespoon low-sodium soy sauce
½ teaspoon ground ginger
1 large clove garlic, crushed
¼ cup low-sodium chicken bouillon
¾ cup sliced mushrooms
¾ cup chopped green beans
½ cup water chestnuts, sliced
½ cup chopped onions
1 small green pepper, cut in chunks
1 8-ounce can unsweetened pineapple chunks,
    juice-packed
1 tablespoon cornstarch
⅜ cup sliced scallions

Combine the sherry, soy sauce, ginger, and garlic in a bowl. Place the chicken cubes in the mixture and marinate in the refrigerator for several hours or overnight.

In a large skillet over high heat, bring the bouillon to a boil. Add the mushrooms and stirfry for a few minutes. Add the green beans, water chestnuts, onions, and green pepper, and stirfry for an additional 2 minutes. Stir in the chicken with the marinade and cook for another 2 minutes.

While the chicken is cooking, drain the pineapple, reserving the juice, and cut the chunks in half, setting them aside. In a small bowl, combine ⅓ cup of the juice with the cornstarch.

Stir this mixture into the skillet with the vegetables and chicken in it, and cook, stirring constantly, until thickened.

Stir in the pineapple and half of the scallions. Garnish with the remaining scallions. This dish is so good with brown rice!
SERVES 2

Roast Chicken à l'Orange

8–10 pieces of chicken, skinned
½ medium onion, minced
1 cup orange juice
½ cup dry white wine
2 tablespoons lemon juice
½ teaspoon dried rosemary, crushed
½ teaspoon dried thyme
½ teaspoon garlic powder
¼ teaspoon paprika
   Freshly ground black pepper to taste
⅛ cup almonds, chopped
½ 4-ounce can mandarin oranges, including liquid

Preheat oven to 400°.

Place chicken pieces, skinned side up, on rack in roasting pan. Add the onion. Then pour half of the orange juice and wine in the pan and sprinkle one tablespoon of lemon juice over the chicken.

In a small bowl, combine all the seasonings and sprinkle half over the chicken. Cover and roast for half an hour.

Turn the chicken. Sprinkle over it the remaining orange juice, wine, lemon juice, and seasonings. Now add the almonds to the pan and, basting occasionally, roast again for 15 minutes.

Pour the mandarin oranges and their liquid over the chicken, place pan under broiler, and broil for 5 minutes. Remove pan from broiler and place chicken pieces on serving platter. Skim and discard any fat from the pan drippings, then pour over chicken and serve.

SERVES 4

Lovers' Chicken

I call this recipe "Lovers' Chicken" because it's so easy—you're free to do anything you want while it's cooking.

    4 pieces chicken (thighs or breasts), skinned
    1 cup white wine
    2 teaspoons garlic powder
    3 tablespoons Cardini's low-cal lemon-lime dressing
        Juice of 1 lemon
    2 teaspoons finely ground black pepper
    ½ teaspoon paprika

Preheat oven to 325°.

Marinate the chicken pieces in the white wine, garlic powder, and lemon-lime dressing for one hour.

Spread the pieces in a casserole and sprinkle fresh lemon juice on top, then spoon marinade over each piece and sprinkle with pepper and paprika. Bake for thirty minutes or until well done. Serve.
SERVES 2–4

Note: For a variation on this dish, you can add baby onions, mushrooms and/or steamed vegetables before baking.

Lemon-Lime Chicken

   4 pieces chicken (thighs or breasts), skinned
   ½ cup Cardini's low-cal lemon-lime dressing
   ½ teaspoon finely ground pepper
   2 teaspoons paprika
   ½ lemon, sliced

With a fork, puncture the chicken pieces three times each. Place in a bowl, pour dressing on top, and cover bowl. Marinate for 20–60 minutes.

Preheat oven to "Broil."

Place the chicken on a cookie-sheet, sprinkle with paprika and pepper, then garnish with lemon. Broil for ten minutes on each side and serve.
SERVES 2

Kim's Chicken Curry

        1 small whole boneless chicken breast, skinned and
            cut into 1-inch cubes
    1¼ cup chicken stock, vegetable stock, or low-sodium
            chicken bouillon
        1 small onion, chopped
        2 carrots, diced
        ½ green or red pepper, chopped
        1 tablespoon canned low-sodium tomato paste
        1 tablespoon low-sodium soy sauce
        ½ teaspoon freshly grated ginger
        ½ teaspoon chili powder
        ½ teaspoon curry powder
        ¼ teaspoon ground cardamom
        ¼ teaspoon turmeric powder
        ⅛ teaspoon cloves
        ½ stick cinnamon, *or* ½ teaspoon ground cinnamon
        1 drop Tabasco (optional)
            Handful of raisins
        1 cup nonfat plain yogurt

    Condiments (optional): an additional ¾ cup nonfat
        yogurt, fresh or canned (unsweetened) pineapple
        chunks

In a large skillet, bring ¼ cup of the stock or bouillon to a boil. Add the chicken, onion, carrots, and chopped pepper, and cook over medium heat 3–5 minutes.

Stir in the remaining stock and the other ingredients, and bring to a boil. Lower heat and simmer, uncovered, until the vegetables are tender. Remove the cinnamon stick, stir in yo-

gurt, and serve hot, spooned over brown rice. Have the diners help themselves individually to the condiments.
SERVES 3

Chicken-stuffed Green Peppers

½ pound ground chicken (no skin)
2 large green peppers
1 tablespoon unsalted margarine
2 tablespoons chopped celery
1 tablespoon chopped onion
½ cup cooked brown rice
1 small tomato, chopped
    Freshly ground black pepper to taste
1 4-ounce can (½ cup) plus 2 tablespoons tomato
    sauce
½ teaspoon raw sugar
¼ teaspoon chopped fresh basil
1 tablespoon grated Parmesan cheese

Preheat oven to 350°.

Cut tops from the peppers; remove the insides. Place peppers in a large saucepan, pour in enough water to cover, and bring to a boil; lower heat and simmer for 5 minutes. Drain and set aside.

In large skillet, melt the margarine and brown the chicken, celery, and onion; drain the excess fat. Add the rice, tomato, pepper, and 2 tablespoons of the tomato sauce and mix well. Spoon the mixture into the peppers, then place them into a shallow baking pan (use tongs if you can).

In a small bowl, combine the remaining ½ cup tomato sauce, sugar, and basil; mix well. Spoon half of the sauce over the

peppers. Bake uncovered for 40 minutes or until the peppers are tender. Spoon on the rest of the sauce, sprinkle with the Parmesan, and bake 5 minutes longer. Serve.
SERVES 2

Teriyaki Chicken

1–1½ pounds boneless chicken, skinned and cut into
1–1½-inch cubes
2 tablespoons chopped scallion
½ tablespoon raw sugar or artificial sweetener
¼ teaspoon ground ginger
2 garlic cloves, minced
½ cup low-sodium soy sauce
⅛ cup dry sherry
1 green or red pepper, cut into 1-inch squares
12 button mushrooms, left whole
8 small white onions
8 cherry tomatoes

4–6 skewers

Preheat oven to "Broil."

In a medium bowl, combine all the ingredients except for the chicken, and mix well. Then add the chicken and stir to coat well. Cover and let stand for 2 hours in the refrigerator. If you remember, stir the chicken occasionally to keep it coated.

On skewers, alternate the chicken with the peppers, mushrooms, onions, and tomatoes, and broil 3–4 inches from the heat in a glass baking dish until the meat is the way you like it. Serve with rice.
SERVES 3

Chicken or Turkey Tacos

⅛ cup chicken stock, vegetable stock, or low-sodium
    bouillon
½ cup finely chopped onion
½ cup finely chopped green or red bell pepper
½ 4-ounce can diced green chiles
½ tablespoon finely chopped seeded jalapeño chile
 1 cup diced cooked chicken or turkey
 1 teaspoon low-sodium soy sauce
¾ teaspoon dried basil
½ teaspoon garlic powder
   Dash cayenne pepper
 6 taco shells

   Raw vegetable garnishes: shredded lettuce, diced
       tomatoes, and chopped scallions
   Nonfat plain yogurt or hot sauce for topping

In a skillet, bring the stock to a boil and add the chopped onion
and bell pepper. Sauté the vegetables over medium heat until
softened, 5–7 minutes. Add the chiles, chicken or turkey, and
seasonings; stir well, cover, and cook over medium heat for 4–
5 minutes, or until thoroughly heated.

Spoon ⅓ cup of the filling into each taco shell. Add the raw-
vegetable garnishes and a dollop of nonfat yogurt. If you like
your taco hot, add a drop of bottled hot sauce.
MAKES 6 tacos (2–4 servings).

Chicken with White Wine and Tarragon

　　1 whole fresh frying chicken
　　　Freshly ground black pepper to taste
　　　Twist of lemon peel
　½ teaspoon dried tarragon
　　1 cup water
　　2 tablespoons unsalted margarine
　　2 tablespoons flour
　½ cup dry white wine
　　2 teaspoons Dijon mustard

Preheat oven to 425°.

Sprinkle the chicken with pepper. Tuck the twist of lemon peel and sprinkle ¼ teaspoon of the tarragon inside the chicken. Place in a roasting pan, pour in 1 cup water, and cover the tin loosely with foil. Bake for 1¼ to 1½ hours, or until cooked. Remove from the oven, remove skin from the chicken, and cut into serving pieces. Lay the pieces on a hot dish and cover to keep warm while you make the sauce.

Strain the juices left in the roasting pan and set aside. Melt the margarine in a saucepan. Stir in the flour and cook for 1 minute. Gradually stir in the strained pan-juices, then add the white wine. Bring to a boil, stirring constantly, and add the mustard and remaining ¼ teaspoon of tarragon. Simmer, stirring, for a few mintues. Pour over the chicken and serve immediately.

SERVES 6

Roast Chicken With Tarragon

1 3½-pound roasting chicken
Freshly ground black pepper to taste
½ teaspoon dried tarragon, *or* 1 teaspoon chopped,
   fresh tarragon
Twist of lemon peel
Flour, to thicken gravy
Dash white wine or lemon juice

Preheat your oven to 400°.

Remove the giblets from the chicken. Sprinkle the inside of the chicken with pepper and a little tarragon, then place the twist of lemon peel inside. Scatter some more tarragon and pepper over the outside. Place the chicken in a roasting pan. Add 1 cup hot water to the pan, cover it loosely with foil, and cook for about 1¼ hours. While it's cooking, check occasionally to make sure that the liquid in the pan has not dried out —be sure to add a little more water if it looks low.

When the chicken is ready, the juice that runs from it should be clear and not pink. Lift it to a hot carving dish. Pour off any fat from the pan-juices and thicken with a little flour moistened in cold water; then add a dash of white wine or a squeeze of lemon juice, according to taste. Remove the skin from the chicken, strain the gravy, and serve.
SERVES 4–6

Roast Breast of Turkey

> 1 2½- to 3-pound turkey breast
> 1 stalk celery with leaves, chopped
> ½ onion, chopped
> 2 tomatoes, chopped
> 2 zucchini, chopped
> ¼ teaspoon garlic powder
> Ground sage, to taste
> ¼–½ teaspoon poultry seasoning (low-sodium if
>   possible)
> ⅔ cup water

Preheat oven to 375°.

Place chopped vegetables in a large baking pan to make a "bed" for the turkey.

Remove the skin and any visible fat from the turkey and rub the breast meat with the seasonings. Place the turkey on the bed of vegetables and add ¾ cup of water to the pan. Cover the pan with aluminum foil and place in the oven for 1¾–2¾ hours. Baste the turkey with the pan-juices every half-hour and if necessary add a little more water. Test for doneness by inserting a fork into the meat. When done, the meat will be tender and the juices will run clear, not pink. Do not overcook.

Remove the cooked turkey breast from the oven and let it stand for about 10 minutes before slicing.

SERVES 6

Note: Turkey is delicious, hot or cold—reserve the leftover and serve sliced, cold.

Apple Turkey Breast

  1 4- to 5-pound turkey breast
  ½ cup unsalted margarine
  1 cup apple juice
    Pinch salt
  3 cloves garlic, peeled and mashed
  ¼ teaspoon paprika

Preheat oven to 325°.

Put the turkey breast on a rack in a roasting pan. Roast in the oven for about an hour.

In a small saucepan melt the margarine: mix in the apple juice, salt, garlic, and paprika. Baste the turkey with the mixture every 15 minutes or so.

When the turkey is done, gently remove the skin and slice the meat into ½-inch slices. Put the slices on a platter and surround them with the Carrots in Lemon Cups (see p. 196). On an adjacent platter, I serve baked potatoes. Another good side dish with this is my Honey Apples (see p. 211).
SERVES 8–10

FISH AND SHELLFISH

Portuguese-style Halibut

2 fresh halibut steaks, 1–1¼ inches thick
Pepper to taste
4 small white onions
1 tomato, peeled, seeded, and chopped, *or* 1 16-
ounce can low-sodium tomatoes, seeded and
chopped
1 clove garlic, finely chopped
1 green pepper
1 red pepper
1 teaspoon dried thyme
1 teaspoon dried rosemary
⅓ cup dry white wine

Preheat broiler.

Wash and dry the fish, and sprinkle with pepper on both sides. Set slices on the broiler pan and broil for 2 minutes on each side. Set aside.

In a nonstick skillet, gently cook the onions until golden (you can use a little margarine or Pam, if you wish, to ensure the onions won't burn); set aside on a plate. In the same skillet, cook the chopped tomatoes and the garlic for a few minutes.

Meanwhile, cut the peppers into thin strips, put them under the broiler, and char on both sides. Place in a bowl of cold water with ice, then peel skin off easily.

Put the onions, tomatoes, and peppers into a saucepan. Add the thyme, rosemary, and white wine. Mix well and bring to a boil. Add the fish steaks to the pan and spoon some of the vegetables over them. Cover, reduce heat, and simmer for 12–15 minutes.

Remove the steaks to a platter; keep them warm. Bring the sauce to a high boil and reduce for 3–4 minutes to blend the flavors well. Spoon over the fish and serve.
SERVES 2

Grilled Swordfish

> 2 swordfish steaks, 1 inch thick, *or* 2 salmon or
> halibut steaks
> 2 tablespoons unsalted margarine, melted
> 1 tablespoon lemon juice
> ½ cup plain nonfat yogurt
> ½ tablespoon chopped fresh dill, *or* ¼ teaspoon dried

Preheat broiler.

Combine the margarine and lemon juice. Broil the fish 5 minutes per side, first brushing each side with the lemon-margarine mixture.

In a blender or food processor, cream the yogurt for 5 seconds, then mix in the dill by hand. When the fish is done, top with the dill-yogurt mixture and serve.
SERVES 2

Salmon Sauté with Fresh Vegetables

> 4 salmon steaks
> Pepper to taste
> 2 tablespoons unsalted butter or margarine
> ¼ cup chopped scallions
> ¼ teaspoon dried thyme
> 1½ cups sliced zucchini
> 1½ cups sliced mushrooms
> ¼ cup water
> 1 teaspoon grated lemon peel
> 4–6 lemon slices

In a skillet, heat 1 tablespoon butter. Add scallions and thyme, and sauté 30 seconds. Stir in zucchini, mushrooms, water, and lemon peel. Simmer over medium heat, covered, until the vegetables are tender, about 15 minutes.

While vegetables are cooking, season salmon with pepper. In a separate skillet, sauté salmon in 1 tablespoon butter over medium heat until browned on both sides (about 10 minutes).

Put salmon on a serving plate. Cover with the vegetables, garnish with lemon slices, and serve.

SERVES 4

Baked Salmon with Cucumber Sauce

            2 salmon steaks
            2 tablespoons melted unsalted margarine
                Ground pepper to taste
        ½ cup nonfat plain yogurt
        1 teaspoon chopped fresh parsley
        ¼ teaspoon chopped fresh chives
        4 tablespoons finely chopped, peeled cucumber
        ½ teaspoon lemon juice

Heat oven to 350°.

Place salmon in greased shallow baking pan; brush with margarine and season with pepper. Bake uncovered for 30–40 minutes or until the fish flakes easily.

In a small bowl, mix together the remaining ingredients; pour over the salmon. Return salmon to oven for another 5 minutes. Remove from oven and place salmon on a serving platter, pouring any leftover pan-juices over the fish. Serve.
SERVES 2–4

Note: This sauce is just as delicious over other fish, such as swordfish, halibut, and sole.

Baked Cod Stew

> 1 pound cod fillets
> ½ tablespoon low-sodium beef bouillon
>   Freshly ground black pepper to taste
> 1 tablespoon lemon juice
> ¼ cup dry white wine
> 1 tablespoon unsalted margarine
> 2 scallions, chopped
> 1 carrot, scraped and diced
> 1 medium onion, chopped
> 1 pound green beans, cut into 1-inch lengths and
>   steamed
> 1 tomato, chopped
> 1 tablespoon raisins
> ½ teaspoon sugar
> ½ tablespoon red wine vinegar
> ½ tablespoon chopped fresh parsley

Preheat oven to 350°.

Place the fish fillets in an ovenproof casserole. Season the fish with bouillon and pepper, and pour lemon juice and wine into the casserole. Bake for 15 minutes.

While the cod is baking, melt the margarine in a large skillet. Add the scallions, carrot, and onion. Cook over very low heat for ten minutes, stirring occasionally. Then stir in green beans, tomato, and raisins. Cook 5 minutes more. Stir in the sugar and vinegar, and then pour the whole mixture over the fish and bake for another 20 minutes. Remove from oven, sprinkle with parsley, and serve.

SERVES 4

Soul Sole

   4 sole fillets, 1–1½ pounds fish altogether
   1 teaspoon paprika
   2 teaspoons chopped fresh dill, *or* ½ teaspoon dried
   1 teaspoon garlic powder
      Black pepper to taste
   2 tablespoons capers
½ red onion, thinly sliced

   4 large squares aluminum foil

Preheat oven to 325°.

Place each fillet on a square of foil. Sprinkle half the paprika, dill, garlic powder, and pepper on the fish, turn over gently, and sprinkle the rest on the other side. Garnish each fillet with red onion slices and sprinkled capers. Wrap each fillet in its own foil "sack," place on a cookie sheet, and bake for 20 minutes or until flaky. Serve still in sacks, to be cut open by each diner at the table.
SERVES 2

Sole Salsa Victoria

   4 sole or sea bass fillets, 1–1½ pounds fish altogether
   1 teaspoon paprika
      Coarsely ground black pepper to taste
   1 teaspoon garlic powder
   4 pickled cherry peppers

   4 large squares aluminum foil

Preheat oven to 325°.

Place each fillet on a square of foil. Sprinkle half the paprika, black pepper, and garlic powder on the fillets; turn the fish over and sprinkle the rest on the other side. Slice the cherry peppers and spread the slices, juice, and seeds over each fillet. Wrap each fillet in a foil "sack," place on cookie sheet, and bake for 20 minutes. Serve.

SERVES 2

Note: For spicier fish, use more cherry peppers.

Cheese-stuffed Trout

    1 tablespoon of flour
    1 1-pound whole trout, cleaned
    ¼ cup sliced fresh mushrooms
    ⅛ cup chopped scallions
    1 tablespoon grated Parmesan cheese
      White or black pepper to taste

In a small bowl, combine mushrooms, scallions, and cheese; spoon mixture into cavity of the fish. Fasten the fish with toothpicks or skewers to keep the stuffing inside. Season with pepper. Place on lightly greased broiler pan. Broil 4 to 5 inches from the heat, 5–10 minutes on each side or until the fish flakes easily.

You can use fish fillets instead of a whole fish. First coat the fillets with flour and season with pepper. In a large skillet, sauté the mushrooms and scallions in small amount of oil until slightly tender. Add the fillets and fry until the fish flakes.

Serve fillets topped with mushrooms and scallions; sprinkle with Parmesan cheese, and serve.
SERVES 2–4

Snapper and Peppers

½ pound red snapper fillets
½ tablespoon oil
1 green pepper, chopped
2 cloves garlic, minced
⅛ teaspoon cinnamon
1 bay leaf
⅛ teaspoon ground coriander
   Pinch cayenne pepper
½ teaspoon turmeric
½ can (3 ounces) low-sodium tomato paste
1 tablespoon lemon juice
1 carrot, scraped, cut into 1" "coins" and boiled
½ tablespoon low-sodium chicken bouillon

Preheat oven to "Broil."

In a medium skillet, heat oil and stir-fry green pepper over low heat for 5 minutes. Add the garlic, cinnamon, bay leaf, coriander, cayenne, turmeric, and tomato paste. Stirfry for one minute.

Place fillets in a shallow pan and sprinkle with lemon juice. Sprinkle carrots around fillets, then sprinkle bouillon on the fish and pour the green pepper and sauce over it all. Broil fillets for 6 minutes on each side, basting often with sauce. Remove to platter and serve.
SERVES 2

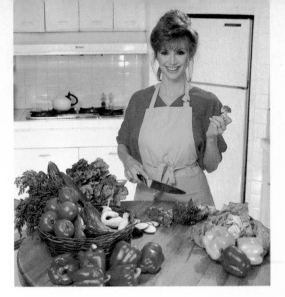

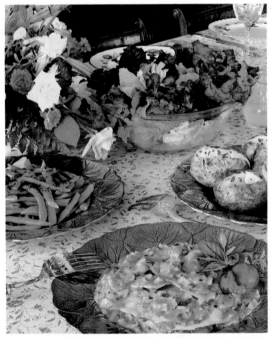

◁ *Veal with Side Dishes*

Sometimes when I have a couple of friends over for dinner, I prefer to put the food out on the table, buffet style. There are two reasons for this—people can then help themselves to as much or as little food as they prefer and I don't have to jump up and down to serve anyone. For this dinner party, I made my Veal Scallops in Tomato Sauce, baked potatoes with Yogurt Dressing, fresh green beans dressed with lemon, and a simple green salad with a vinaigrette dressing. It is a delicious and nutritious meal that looks pretty and elegant!

Chinese Sesame-Chicken Salad ▷

My Chinese Sesame-Chicken Salad is a simple lunch dish or a wonderful appetizer to begin a meal. Just set it on an elegant black plate or on porcelain with a more elaborate Chinese design, add colorful napkins, chopsticks and flowers, and the mood is set. That's important—it ensures that what could have been a boring chicken salad becomes an inviting dish anytime.

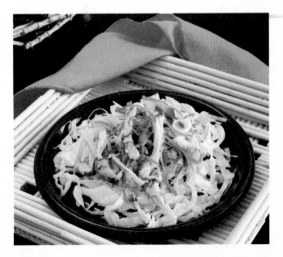

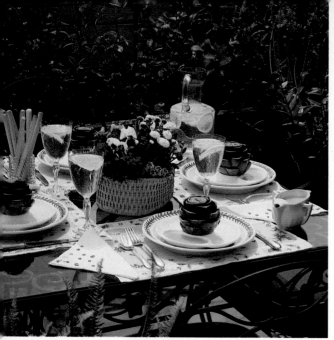

◁ Artichokes

I love artichokes! They are full of potassium and Vitamin A, they taste great and always look so special on a table. They are also easy to make—I cook mine in water with basil and lemon and serve them with a side sauce of yogurt or mustard. This pretty setting in the garden was the beginning of a lunch for some friends visiting from out of town. The fresh linen napkins, the flowers in a basket, and the outdoor atmosphere really help to make an easy lunch memorable.

Strawberries in Bed ▽

Here is a breakfast guaranteed to make you start your day with a smile! Easy to prepare, healthful to eat, luxuriously served on a simple bed tray, it ensures a lovely beginning to your day.

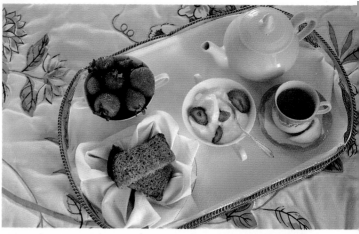

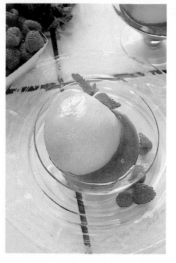

Peaches in Raspberry Sauce △

Talk about simple and gorgeous! Peaches make enticing desserts that are always a big hit.

Spaghettini with Asparagus ▷

Dinner for two—even this simple pasta looks like a feast for kings! And it tastes wonderful—and doesn't look like a meal you eat on a diet, does it?

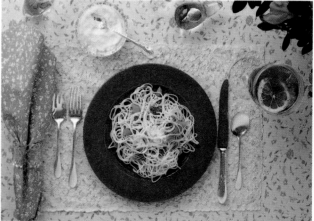

Chicken Kabobs   ▷

Chicken Kabobs are a staple in my life—easy to make, healthful and delicious to eat, and lovely to serve. Also a terrific last-minute meal—for yourself and for unexpected company.

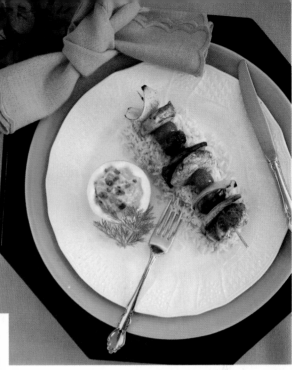

Bread Basket   ▽

I love bread! Bread in some form is an integral part of all my diets—an important nutritional supplement, so don't leave it out of your diet and think you are doing yourself a favor. You need the nutrition good bread provides.

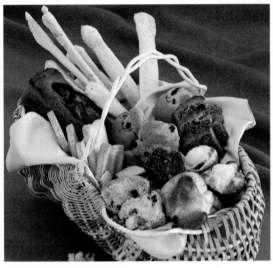

Trifle   ▷

Many of my guests exclaim in surprise when served my delicious trifle. I guess it doesn't seem that I would eat such a "rich" dessert. But as you already know, I am not in favor of abstaining from wonderful desserts for the rest of my life—so a trifle now and then won't hurt you. And what's more, my trifle is made with a minimum of "problematic" ingredients. So enjoy!

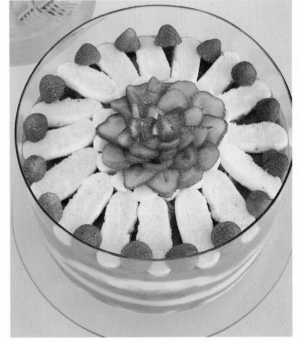

Salmon Mousse ◁

Beautiful and tasty! What more can you ask? It's good for you, too. I serve this for dinner for two or for twenty. Salmon is a very nutritious fish, and when made into a mousse it is as elegant as it is good. The added plus is that it's easy to make!

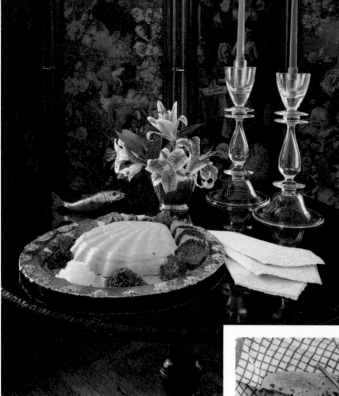

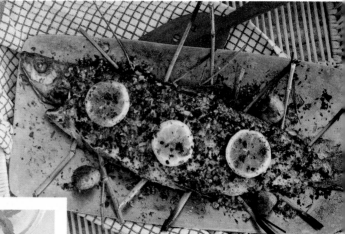

Cheese-stuffed Trout △

I love this dish! It tastes terrific and looks so impressive when I serve it. I first learned to make it in England and have been serving it ever since.

◁ *Baked Salmon with Cucumber Sauce*

As salmon and chicken are perfect sources of calcium and protein, I have developed many variations of both. The baked salmon steak is the easiest to prepare—I particularly like it with a cucumber sauce (made with yogurt) poured over it.

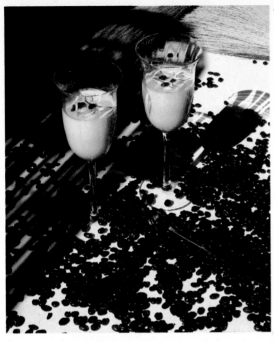

Coffee Smoothies

Easy, delicious, and gorgeous! What more can you ask for? Serve this to your guests for any summer lunch or dinner and they'll be singing your praises!

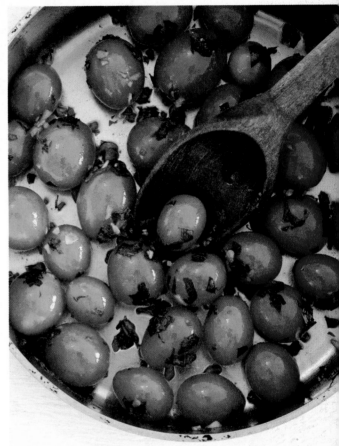

Sautéed Cherry Tomatoes ▷

This is a simple way to make tomatoes—just throw them in a pan, sauté, sprinkle with fresh basil, and serve.

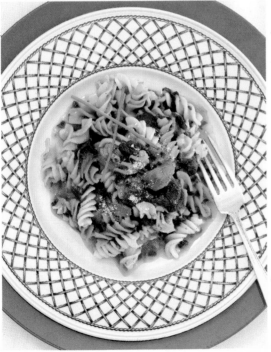

◁ Corkscrew Pasta with Spinach

You don't have to be part Italian to love pasta—any shape, with any sauce. This is a particular favorite of mine—an easy dish to make for friends or just for yourself.

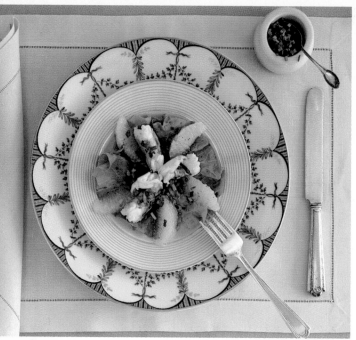

◁Shrimp and Orange Salad

I'll bet you never thought of this combination, but I've been marrying shrimp and oranges for years. The taste of the two is a perfect combination your taste buds will adore! They also make a beautiful and colorful dish.

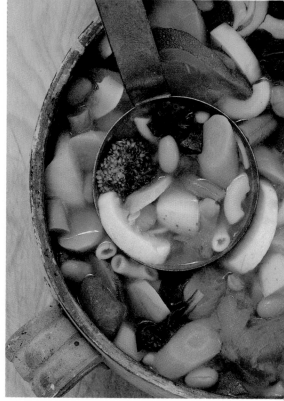

Vegetable Minestrone Soup ▷

This is one of my favorite winter soups—you can make it one day, serve it the next, freeze the remainder, and then blend it to make a wonderful ''cream of vegetable'' soup. Your friends will be sure to ask for this recipe—so tell them to buy the book!

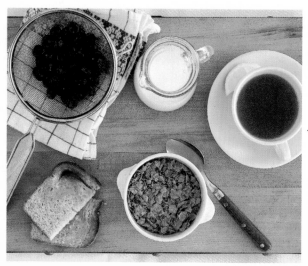

◁Breakfast with Blueberries!

Any berries make a nutritious and delicious addition to your breakfast tray. Serve them on cereal, covered with yogurt, or simply in a bowl. The trick is to make sure the berries are fresh—check with your market and you may be surprised at the variety of berries that are in season at various times of the year.

Salade Niçoise ▷

My variation on an old theme—I love this salad and could live on it! I often eat it in my dressing room on my lunch hour. It's easy to make and always filling.

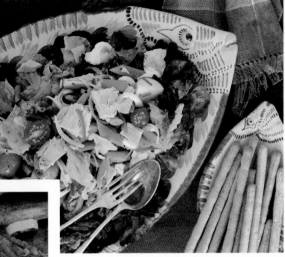

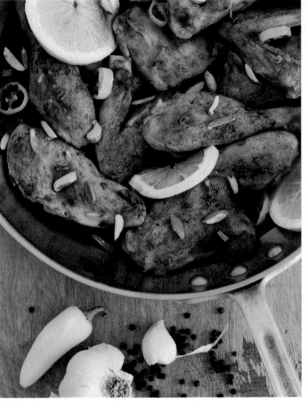

◁ Chicken Vera Cruz

The combination of ingredients in this super dish—oranges, peanuts, chilies—makes it unforgettable. This is no ordinary chicken—make it once and you'll definitely make it again.

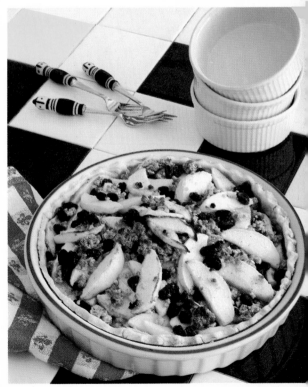

Apple Pie ▷

Fresh, hot steaming, cinnamony—right out of the oven. Everything in it is good for you. Everything in it will make your mouth water. It is so simple to make—give yourself a treat! Don't wait for company—make it just for yourself!

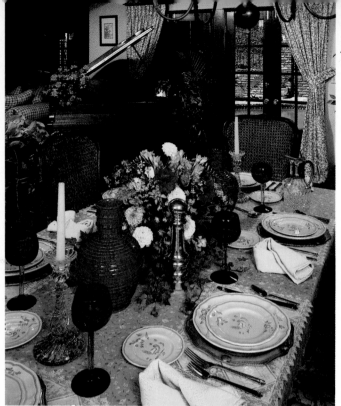

◁ Victoria's Dining Table

This is my dining room set for a dinner party. I love my table to look somehow casual, yet lovely. I don't feel a need to impress my friends with a lot of formal silver and china. I prefer simplicity, and a lot of warmth. Now all we need is the food!

Iced Tea ▽

I live on iced tea! Summer or winter, I find it the perfect drink. It satisfies my thirst, fulfills my requirements of drinking a lot of liquid every day, and is delicious. Make it with lemons, oranges, and a bit of mint, and you may never drink soft drinks again!

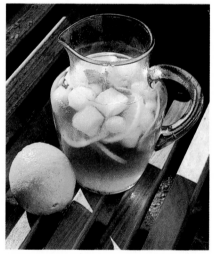

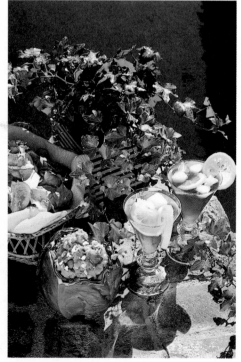

◁ Green Bean Guacamole, Tea and Chips

Let them think it's avocados! Then surprise them—it's a guacamole made from green beans! No unwanted fat here—just a delicious appetizer or snack. Add the tea and homemade potato chips and you're in business.

Easy Baked Fish in Sauce

    3 ¼-pound fish fillets (cod, halibut, salmon, sole
        swordfish, haddock, etc.)
    ¼ cup dry white wine
    2 tablespoons orange juice
    1 tablespooon lemon juice
    ½ teaspoon low-sodium soy sauce
    ½ tablespoon chopped fresh dill, *or* ¼ teaspoon dried
    ½ teaspoon onion powder
        Freshly ground black pepper to taste
    ¼ cup chopped scallions
    2 tablespoons chopped fresh parsley
    1 lemon, sliced

Preheat oven to 450°

Arrange the fillets in a baking dish. In a small bowl, mix together the other ingredients, except the scallions, parsley, and
lemon slices, and pour over the fillets; sprinkle with the scallions. Cover the dish and bake in the oven for 25 minutes.
Transfer the fish and sauce to a serving dish. Garnish with
lemon slices and parsley, and serve.
SERVES 2–3

Baked Fish Pernod

1 large (2–3 pound) fillet of sea bass or white fish
3 medium onions, finely chopped
2 cloves garlic, finely chopped
2 tablespoons finely chopped fresh parsley
2 tablespoons finely chopped fresh chervil
2 tablespoons finely chopped fresh tarragon
½ cup dry white wine
½ cup water
2 tablespoons Pernod (or other anise-flavored liquor)
1 large lemon, thinly sliced
2 tablespoons margarine
   Freshly ground black pepper to taste

Preheat oven to 450°.

In a small bowl, combine the onions, garlic, parsley, chervil, tarragon, wine, water, and Pernod. Place the fish in a large baking dish, and pour the mixture over it. Cover with lemon slices, dot with margarine, and season with pepper.

Bake for 30–40 minutes (or until the fish flakes easily with a fork), basting from time to time. If fish becomes too dry, add a little more water and wine. When done, remove fish to serving platter, pour remaining sauce over it, and serve.
SERVES 2–4

Note: To give this dish a sophisticated look, place dried fennel leaves (available in specialty stores) on your serving tray and lay the fish on the leaves.

Baked Fish with Plum Tomatoes

   ½–1 pound halibut, sea bass, or cod (not rock cod)
         fillets, about 1" thick, cut into 2–4 serving
         pieces
   1 teaspoon Dijon mustard
   2 tablespoons whole wheat flour
   ½ tablespoon paprika
   ½ tablespoon chopped fresh dill, *or* ¼ teaspoon
         dried

SAUCE:
   1 tablespoon dry white wine
   ¼ large onion, chopped
   1 clove garlic, minced or crushed
   ¼ cup finely chopped fresh parsley
   1 28-ounce can whole Italian plum tomatoes,
         drained
   1 cup sliced mushrooms
   1 tablespoon chopped fresh basil, *or* ½ teaspoon
         dried
   1 bay leaf
   1 teaspoon frozen orange-juice concentrate
   1 tablespoon capers

Preheat oven to 350°.

To make the sauce, place the wine in a heated skillet. Add the onion, garlic, and parsley, and sauté over moderate heat for a few minutes, stirring frequently.

Add the tomatoes, mushrooms, basil, bay leaf, and orange juice to the skillet, and simmer, stirring occasionally, for 5 minutes. Remove half of the tomatoes from the skillet and arrange them around the sides of a baking dish. Place the other tomatoes in a blender to purée; then return the puréed tomatoes to the skillet. Stir in the capers. Pour the sauce over the bottom of the baking dish.

Spread the mustard over one side of the fillets. In a shallow bowl, combine the flour, paprika, and dill; dip each fillet in the mixture, coating both sides. Place the fillets (mustard side up) over the sauce in the baking dish, but do not cover with sauce. Cover the baking dish with aluminum foil and bake for 35–40 minutes. When done, remove fish to platter, pour remaining pan-juices over fish, and serve.
SERVES 2–4

Cioppino

> ¾ pound striped or sea bass
> ½ pound raw shrimp
> ¾ pound Dungeness crab with shells, *or* any other
>   fish you prefer
> 1 can clams, oysters, or mussels, drained
> 1 clove garlic, minced
> 1 medium onion, chopped
> 1 green pepper, diced
> 2 tablespoons minced fresh parsley
> 1 cup dry wine, preferably red
> 1¼ cup canned Italian-style plum tomatoes, drained
> 2 tablespoons low-sodium tomato paste
> 1 tablespoon freshly ground black pepper
> ½ teaspoon dried basil
>   Chopped fresh parsley for garnish

Cut the bass into 2-inch square pieces. Shell and devein the shrimp, but leave the tails intact. Cut the crab or other fish into bite-sized pieces.

In a large pot over medium heat, sauté the garlic, onion, green pepper, and 1 tablespoon of the parsley in 2 tablespoons of the wine until the onions are translucent. Chop the tomatoes and add them to the mixture with the rest of the parsley, wine, tomato paste, and seasonings; simmer over low heat for 20 minutes.

Add the fish, shrimp, and other seafood, and cook over low heat for 1 hour. Serve hot with additional chopped parsley as garnish.

SERVES 3–4

Note: Sometimes I add ½ teaspoon dried oregano, but it does give the fish a different flavor—try it both ways.

Fillet Almondine

    2–4 fish fillets, 1–1½ pounds altogether (use just about any fish: salmon, halibut, swordfish, cod, etc.)
    ⅛ cup slivered or sliced almonds
    2 tablespoons unsalted margarine
    ¼ teaspoon garlic powder
    Pepper to taste
    ⅛ teaspoon dried dill
    ½ tablespoon lemon juice

In a large skillet, sauté the almonds in margarine until golden. Remove from pan and set aside. Add fish fillets to pan; season with garlic powder, pepper, and dill; and fry over medium heat until golden brown on both sides and fish flakes easily (don't turn the fish over more than once). Remove to a serving platter. Heat lemon juice and sautéed almonds in the pan drippings, pour over the fish, and serve.

SERVES 2

VARIATION:
For Fillets in Wine-Margarine, add 1 tablespoon white wine or sherry and ¼ teaspoon dried dill when adding lemon juice to pan drippings.

Fish Fillets in White Wine

> 4 small cod, snapper, or salmon fillets, about ¼
>   pound each
> Pinch pepper
> 1 tablespoon lemon juice
> ½ teaspoon garlic powder
> 2 teaspoons low-sodium chicken bouillon
> 3 scallions, chopped
> 2 tablespoons unsalted margarine, melted
> ½ cup dry white wine
> 1 tablespoon chopped fresh parsley
> ½ teaspoon dried thyme
> Pinch cayenne pepper
> 2 bay leaves, crushed
> 1 tablespoon whole wheat flour
> ⅛ cup nonfat plain yogurt

Preheat oven to 375°.

Wash and dry the fillets and arrange in a greased ovenproof casserole in a single layer. Sprinkle with pepper, lemon juice, garlic powder, bouillon, scallions, margarine, wine, parsley, thyme, cayenne, and bay leaves. Cover the casserole, and bake for 20 minutes.

When done, remove the fillets to a warm serving platter. Strain the pan-juices into a saucepan, add the flour, and stir until blended. Add the yogurt and cook, stirring, over medium heat for another 5 minutes. Pour sauce over the fish and serve.

SERVES 4

Fish Creole

    4 fish fillets
    1 tablespoon unsalted margarine
    2 tablespoons finely chopped green pepper
    1 small onion, chopped
    ½ stalk celery, chopped
    2 tablespoons brown sugar, *or* ½ teaspoon liquid
        artificial sweetener
    ¼ teaspoon dried oregano leaves
        Ground pepper to taste
    1 cup low-sodium stewed tomatoes, cut into pieces

Heat oven to 350°.

Arrange fillets in a glass baking dish greased lightly with margarine. In a medium skillet over medium heat, melt the margarine and cook the green pepper, onion, and celery until tender. Stir in remaining ingredients; mix well. Pour mixture over fillets. Bake uncovered for 30–35 minutes or until fish flakes easily.

SERVES 3–4

Poached Fish with Vegetables

1 pound rainbow trout or sea bass fillets
½ teaspoon dried sage
4 teaspoons low-sodium beef bouillon
1 teaspoon dried tarragon
1 teaspoon chopped fresh parsley
1 teaspoon dried basil
¼ cup sweet vermouth
¼ cup dry vermouth
6 scallions, chopped
1 zucchini, thinly sliced
1 pound green beans
2 tablespoons lemon juice
Freshly ground black pepper to taste

Preheat oven to 375°.

Place fillets in a casserole, one layer thick. Sprinkle with sage, bouillon, tarragon, parsley, and basil. Pour vermouth around the fillets and place vegetables over and around them. Add lemon juice over it all, and season with pepper. Cover the casserole and bake for 20 minutes. Serve.
SERVES 2

Fish with Yogurt and Chives

4 sea bass or whitefish fillets, about ¼ pound each
2 tablespoons flour
1 cup nonfat plain yogurt
3 tablespoons chopped fresh chives

Preheat broiler.

Dust the fillets with the flour, place in a greased, glass baking dish, and broil on each side until cooked through, 3–5 minutes. In a small bowl mix the yogurt and chives, and pour over the fish. Put fish back under broiler for 2 minutes, then serve at once. Plain boiled potatoes or brown rice are a good accompaniment.

SERVES 4

Fruited Fish Fillets

Despite the surprising ingredients, this is truly a delicious dish!

> 2 fish fillets (use sole, red snapper, bass, or other lean white fish)
> ¼ cup bottled white grape juice
> ⅛ cup orange juice
> ½ tablespoon lemon juice
> 1 tablespoon white wine
> ½ teaspoon low-sodium soy sauce
> ¼ teaspoon ground ginger
> ¾ teaspoon cornstarch
> ½ teaspoon onion powder
> ¼ teaspoon curry powder
> Pinch cayenne pepper
> ¼ orange, cut into thin, lengthwise wedges

Preheat oven to 375°.

Put the fish in a greased baking dish. In a small bowl, mix half the grape juice with the other fruit juices, wine, soy sauce, and ginger, and pour the mixture over the fish. Cover the baking dish and bake for 15 minutes. Remove cover, baste fish with the juices, and continue baking uncovered 10–15 minutes longer, or until the fish flakes easily with a fork.

Remove the fish from the oven. Leaving the fillets in the dish and taking care not to break them, pour off the pan-juices into a saucepan. Add the remaining grape juice, cornstarch, and spices to the pan-juices. Heat to a boil, and cook until thick. Pour the sauce over the fish fillets, then arrange the orange wedges between and around the fillets.

Return the fish to the oven for 2–3 minutes more. Serve.
SERVES 2

Marinated Bass Teriyaki

        4 bass fillets, about ¼ pound each
        2 tablespoons low-sodium soy sauce
        2 tablespoons water
        1 tablespoon plus 1 teaspoon dry sherry
        1 clove garlic, minced
        ¼ teaspoon ground ginger

In a small bowl, combine soy sauce, water, sherry, garlic, and ginger. Arrange the fillets in an 8"- × -8" buttered glass baking dish and pour the teriyaki mixture over them. Turn the fish over to coat the other side.

Cover dish and refrigerate for 1 hour. Microwave marinated fillets, uncovered, on "High" until fish flakes easily when tested with a fork, 4–5 minutes. Or bake them in the oven for 20 minutes at 350°. Remove fillets to platter, pour sauce over them, and serve.
SERVES 2

Seviche

½ pound bay or sea scallops
½ cup fresh lime juice
1 tablespoon minced onion
½ teaspoon chopped fresh parsley
1 tablespoon chopped green pepper
1 tablespoon unsalted margarine, melted
Ground pepper to taste

Place scallops in a glass bowl. Cover with lime juice and refrigerate at least 12 hours. Turn occasionally. Scallops will "cook" in lime juice, losing their translucent look and becoming firm and white.

Toss with remaining ingredients and serve on lettuce leaves as an appetizer, or with toothpicks as an hors d'oeuvre.
SERVES 3

Shrimp Curry

4 cups uncooked shrimp, shelled and deveined
1 tablespoon unsalted margarine
2 tablespoons finely chopped onion
2 tablespoons curry powder
½ teaspoon ground ginger
1 yellow chile, sliced
½ cup chicken stock
1 cup coconut milk
1 medium cucumber, peeled and sliced in strips
1 tablespoon lemon juice
Pinch cayenne pepper

In a skillet over medium heat, melt the margarine and sauté the onion. Then stir in the curry, ginger, and chile. Pour the chicken stock over the mixture and simmer for 15 minutes, stirring occasionally.

Now add shrimp, coconut milk, cucumber strips, lemon juice, and cayenne. Simmer another 5 minutes or until the shrimp turn a pretty pink. Serve with brown rice and a papaya half.
SERVES 4–6

Shrimp Jambalaya

    1 cup (4-ounces) uncooked medium shrimp, peeled and deveined
    1 slice bacon, cut into small pieces (trim off fat)
    ¼ cup chopped green pepper
    ½ medium onion, chopped
    1 clove garlic, minced
    ½ cup uncooked brown rice
    ¼ teaspoon chili powder
    ½ teaspoon chopped fresh basil
    1 cube or 1 teaspoon low-sodium chicken bouillon
    ½ bay leaf
    ¾ cup water
    1 8-ounce can low-sodium tomatoes, undrained and chopped

In a large skillet over medium heat, fry bacon until crisp. Add green pepper, onion, and garlic; sauté until tender. Stir in rice, chili powder, basil, bouillon, bay leaf, water, and tomatoes.

Heat to boiling, then reduce heat to low and simmer, covered, for 10 minutes or until rice is almost tender. Add the shrimp and cook, uncovered, for another 10–15 minutes, or until shrimp are firm and pink. Remove bay leaf and serve.
SERVES 2

Shrimp Scampi

> 1 pound uncooked jumbo shrimp, peeled and
>   deveined
> 2 tablespoons unsalted margarine
> 2 tablespoons chopped onions
> 1 clove garlic, minced
> 1 tablespoon finely chopped fresh parsley
> ⅓ cup dry bread crumbs
> 1 lemon, sliced or cut into wedges

Preheat broiler.

In a large broiling pan or skillet over medium heat, melt margarine and sauté onions and garlic until golden, about 2–3 minutes. Add shrimp and cook until pink. Sprinkle with parsley and bread crumbs. Place under broiler, and broil for 4 minutes or until the crumbs are golden brown. Serve garnished with lemon slices or wedges.
SERVES 3

VEAL

Veal Piccata

    2–3 veal scallops, about ½ pound altogether
     ¼ cup flour
     ½ cup low-sodium chicken bouillon
     ½ teaspoon dried oregano
     ⅛ teaspoon dried sage
     ½ teaspoon dried basil
     ⅛ teaspoon dried rosemary, crushed
    1–2 teaspoons Dijon mustard
     1 tablespoon olive oil
     2 tablespoons unsalted margarine
     3 tablespoons marsala wine
     3 tablespoons lemon juice
      Chopped fresh parsley

If your butcher hasn't already pounded your veal scallops, place them on a wooden cutting board, cover with wax paper, and pound with a wooden mallet until they are thin.

In a bowl, combine the flour, chicken bouillon, and all the spices. Spread the mustard on each side of the scallops, then coat them with the flour mixture.

Heat the oil and margarine in a large skillet over medium heat. When the margarine has melted, brown the veal quickly, about 3 minutes on each side. Add the wine and simmer for 5–7 minutes. Add the lemon juice, scraping the bottom of the pan to mix the ingredients together. Remove the meat to a serving platter, sprinkle with the chopped parsley, and pour the sauce over it.

This dish is great with rice and steamed broccoli.
SERVES 2

Note: To make more, just add more pieces of veal—this recipe makes enough for up to 8 scallops.

Veal Scallops in Tomato Sauce

I usually make this dish for a dinner party of 6–8 people.

> 12–14 veal scallops
> 2 tablespoons unsalted margarine
> 2 medium onions, chopped
> 1 teaspoon cornstarch
> ½ cup dry white wine (Madeira or marsala is great)
> 4 cups canned Italian plum tomatoes, drained
> ½ teaspoon chopped fresh basil
> ½ teaspoon crushed fresh rosemary
> 1 teaspoon chopped fresh sage
> ½ teaspoon dried oregano, *or* 1 teaspoon chopped
>   fresh oregano
> 1 tablespoon crushed black pepper
> 1 tablespoon capers

If your butcher hasn't already pounded the veal scallops, spread them on a wooden cutting board, cover with wax paper, and pound them with a wooden mallet or the back of a serving spoon until thin.

In a skillet, melt the margarine and sauté the onions. Remove from pan and brown the scallops quickly, about 2 minutes each side. In a small bowl, mix the cornstarch with 3 table-spoons of the white wine and pour over the scallops. Continue cooking the veal until most of the liquid has evaporated. Remove from the pan and put on a serving platter.

Return onions to the pan. Cut the tomatoes into small pieces, and add to the onions. Add the herbs and pepper and simmer for about 5 mniutes. Add the scallops to the tomato mixture. Spoon the sauce over the scallops, and add the capers. Remove to a platter and serve.

VARIATION:
Sauté ½ pound mushrooms in margarine and wine, and add to the tomato mixture before adding the veal.

Veal Stew

2 pounds stewing veal, cut into 2-inch pieces
Black pepper to taste
¼ cup flour
4 tablespoons unsalted margarine
2 cups chopped onion
4 cloves garlic, finely chopped or pressed
¼ teaspoon celery powder
1 cup dry white wine
1½ cups canned tomatoes, mashed and drained
1 cup low-sodium chicken broth
½ teaspoon dried thyme
1 bay leaf
1 cup sliced carrots
1 pound button mushrooms, whole

Sprinkle veal cubes with pepper and coat with flour.

In a large frying pan over medium heat, melt 2 tablespoons of the margarine and add the veal. Cook for about 15 minutes, making sure you stir the pieces so they brown on all sides (I prefer to do this with a wooden spoon—metal instruments tend to take off some of the flour).

After veal is browned, add the onion, garlic, and celery powder (don't substitute celery salt without being aware that it is indeed salt, while celery powder contains no sodium). Continue cooking for 5 minutes, then add the wine, tomatoes, chicken broth, thyme, and bay leaf. Cover the pan, reduce the heat, and simmer for about half an hour.

In another pan over medium heat, melt the other 2 tablespoons of margarine and add the carrots and the mushrooms. Cook for about 5 minutes, then add to the veal. Cover what is now your entire veal dish and let cook for 15 more minutes. (This is a great time to make brown rice. It tastes terrific with this dish.)

SERVES 4–6

SALADS AND SALAD DRESSINGS

Tabbouleh

This salad is a staple of Middle Eastern cuisine, and it is delicious. I often eat a bowl of tabbouleh with some crackers for lunch. It can stay in the refrigerator for at least a week, and makes a good appetizer for a party.

> 1 cup cracked wheat
> 2 large tomatoes, chopped
> ½ cup chopped scallions
> 2 cups chopped fresh parsley
> 2 tablespoons dried mint
> ¼ cup chopped onion
> ¼ cup olive oil
> ¼ teaspoon low-sodium salt
> ¼ teaspoon black or white pepper
> 1 cup lemon juice

Wash the cracked wheat by putting it in a large bowl, adding enough hot water to cover, and letting it stand for a half hour. Then drain the wheat in a colander.

In a large bowl, combine the wheat, tomatoes, scallions, parsley, mint, and onion. Mix well. Then add the oil, salt, pepper, and lemon juice. Stir the mixture until well blended, then cover and refrigerate until you are ready to serve.

SERVES 4

Sole Salad

This is an easy and delicious salad to make with the leftover sole from any of my sole dishes. It doesn't matter how you made the sole—it will still taste great in this salad.

> 2 cups cooked sole, cut into 1" pieces (make sure it is cold—a warm sole will flake and crumble)
> ¼ cup thinly sliced radishes
> ¼ cup chopped scallions
> ¼ cup chopped red pepper
> ¼ cup chopped green pepper
> 1 cup peeled and thinly sliced cucumber
> 2 tomatoes, cut in chunks
> Butter (Boston) lettuce
> Red lettuce
> Freshly chopped parsley for garnish

In a bowl, mix the sole, radishes, scallions, peppers, cucumbers, and tomatoes, and toss. Add as much or as little lettuce as you like, and then dress with either my Green Goddess Dressing (p. 181), No-Guilt Salad Dressing (p. 180), or Yogurt Dressing (p. 181). Garnish with parsley and serve.
SERVES 4–6

Low-calorie, Low-sodium Vinaigrette Dressing

½ cup olive or other vegetable oil
1¾ teaspoons paprika
1 teaspoon dry mustard
1½ cloves garlic, crushed
½ teaspoon dried basil
⅛ teaspoon black pepper
1 tablespoon chopped onions or chives
3 tablespoons cider or red wine vinegar
2 tablespoons lemon juice
2 teaspoons chopped fresh parsley

Combine all ingredients. Let sit in a covered jar in refrigerator at least 12 hours before serving. Remember to always shake well before using. (Sometimes I put the dressing in my food processor for a few seconds. It blends all the ingredients and results in a smooth dressing.)

No-Guilt Salad Dressing

2 tablespoons rice vinegar
1 teaspoon Dijon mustard
Sweet 'n Low Sweetener to taste

Mix all the ingredients and pour over any salad. You can vary the dressing—for example, add 1 teaspoon chopped chives or 1 teaspoon chopped shallots. But never any cream, OK?

Green Goddess Dressing

1 garlic clove, crushed
3 tablespoons chopped scallions
1 tablespoon lemon juice
3 tablespoons vinegar
1 cup nonfat plain yogurt
½ cup chopped fresh parsley
Black pepper to taste

Blend all the ingredients except for the yogurt in the blender or the food processor for 1 minute. Now add the yogurt and blend for 10 seconds using the start and stop button (if you blend too long the dressing will be too thin). Serve over salad.

Yogurt Dressing

This is a wonderful dressing for salads and it works equally well over cold salmon.

1 cup nonfat plain yogurt
1 teaspoon finely chopped fresh chives
¼ cup finely chopped watercress
1 clove garlic, pressed
½ teaspoon dried dill
½ teaspoon dried tarragon
½ teaspoon Dijon mustard
Pinch pepper
Pinch salt (just this once)
Pinch sugar or artificial sweetener

In your blender or food processor, blend the yogurt until creamy. Put in a jar and add all the other ingredients. Mix with a spoon and refrigerate.
MAKES 1½–2 CUPS

SAUCES

Garlic and Tarragon Sauce for Steamed, Baked, or Poached Fish

Fish fillet of your choice, steamed, baked, or
poached

SAUCE:
1 cup dry white wine
3 teaspoons dried tarragon
3 tablespoons unsalted margarine
2 tablespoons flour
1 clove garlic, crushed
½ cup low-sodium (if possible) chicken stock
Freshly ground black pepper to taste

While your fish fillet is cooking, prepare the sauce. Boil the wine in a saucepan until it is reduced by half. Add the tarragon and let stand.

In another saucepan over medium heat, melt the margarine and stir in the flour. Cook for 1 minute, then add the garlic, stock, and pepper. Bring to a boil, and cook, stirring continually, until the sauce is smooth and thickened. Remove from heat, and stir in the wine and tarragon mixture.

When your fish is ready, strain the sauce and pour over the fish. Serve immediately.

Herb Butter for Basting Fish or Chicken

   2 tablespoons unsalted margarine, softened
   ¼ teaspoon lemon juice
   ⅛ teaspoon dry mustard
   1 tablespoon chopped fresh parsley
   1 tablespoon chopped fresh chives

Mix all the ingredients in a small saucepan, and heat for about 5 minutes. Use this mixture to baste fish or chicken as you bake or broil them.

Garlic Sauce

   2 cloves garlic, crushed
   1 teaspoon dried fine herbs
   2 teaspoons lemon juice
   3 tablespoons low-fat plain yogurt
   ½ teaspoon celery powder

Blend the ingredients in a blender or food processor until smooth (use the start and stop button—don't blend too long or the sauce will become too runny).

Note: This is great as a dip for raw vegetables.

Salsa

> 1 teaspoon vegetable oil
> 2 tablespoons chopped onion
> 2 tablespoons chopped green pepper
> ½ teaspoon chopped green chiles (low-sodium canned are fine)
> 2 cups chopped tomatoes (you can blend in the food processor if you like)
> Pinch garlic powder
> 1 drop Tabasco

In a saucepan over medium heat, heat the oil for 3 minutes, then add the onions, peppers, and chiles and sauté for 5–7 minutes. Then add all the other ingredients and simmer for another 5 minutes.

Remove from heat and let cool. Refrigerate until ready to use. Serve the sauce cold.
SERVES 2

Mustard Sauce

This sauce is just wonderful on hot or cold chicken or fish, and salads.

> 2 tablespoons Dijon mustard
> ½ cup nonfat plain yogurt
> 1 teaspoon vinegar

Blend all the ingredients in your blender or food processor, or beat together with a whisk in a bowl. Put into a small bowl, and refrigerate until ready to use.
MAKES ABOUT 1 CUP

Tomato Sauce

This recipe is so good and so easy that I stopped using ready-made spaghetti sauce years ago.

> 5 pounds ripe plum tomatoes, halved (if your market has Italian tomatoes, use those)
> ½ cup chopped fresh basil
> 5 cloves garlic, peeled and halved
> 2 teaspoons dried oregano
> 1 teaspoon dried rosemary, crushed
> Freshly ground black pepper to taste
> Pinch raw sugar

In a saucepan bring 4 cups of water to a boil. When boiling, throw in the tomatoes, three or four at a time, and leave in for 30–45 seconds. Remove with tongs and peel the skin (it will come off easily). Do this until all the tomatoes have been skinned. Now put the tomatoes in your food processor and chop coarsely.

In another saucepan, combine the chopped tomatoes with all the other ingredients, and cook over a low flame for 35–40 minutes.

Remove the sauce from the pan and let cool. Then spoon over pasta or freeze. With this recipe I always have extra to use again.

Note: When you are using a dried spice, take the desired amount and rub together between the palms of your hands. This will bring out the freshness of the spice. Then simply put into the pot.

PASTA

Corkscrew Pasta with Spinach

Corkscrew pasta, as much as you need—in general, ¼–⅓ pound per person (you can buy tomato, spinach, and/or carrot pasta made with no preservatives)
4 quarts water

SAUCE:
2 tablespoons olive oil
3 cups chopped ripe tomatoes (Italian plum are best), *or* 1 28-ounce can crushed tomatoes
1 package frozen spinach, thawed and drained
  Pinch white pepper
1 tablespoon lemon juice

¼ cup grated Parmesan cheese
2 chives for garnish

Bring the water to a boil and add the pasta. Cook for about 10 minutes, or until it reaches the consistency you prefer. (Feel free to follow the cooking directions on the pasta package.)

While the pasta cooks, heat the olive oil in a skillet over medium heat. Add the tomatoes to the skillet; cook for 3 minutes. Then add the spinach, pepper, and lemon juice, and cook until the pasta is ready.

When the pasta is done, drain, rinse with warm water, and put into a serving bowl, and pour the sauce over it. Top with the cheese and two chives crossed in an "x," and serve.
SERVES 2–4, depending on how much pasta you make.

Note: If you're only serving two people, you'll probably have extra sauce—freeze it.

Herbed Pasta

> Spaghettini for two
> 4 quarts water

> *SAUCE:*
> 1 tablespoon olive oil
> 1 tablespoon unsalted margarine
> 2 tablespoons chopped fresh parsley
> 1 tablespoon chopped fresh basil
> 2 tablespoons chopped fresh chives
> 2–3 clove garlic, peeled and mashed
> ¼ cup grated Parmesan cheese

Bring the water to a boil and add the spaghetti. Cook for about 5 minutes, or until it reaches the consistency you prefer.

Immediately after you add the pasta to the water, melt the oil and margarine in a skillet. Add the parsley, basil, chives, and garlic, and sauté for about 5 minutes.

When the pasta is done, drain and rinse with warm water (to get the excess starch off), and put in a bowl. Pour the sauce over the spaghetti, top with the cheese, and serve.
SERVES 2

Pasta with Vegetables

Pasta of your choice
4 quarts water

SAUCE:
4 ripe tomatoes (Italian plum are best)
2 teaspoons unsalted margarine
¼ teaspoon dried oregano
1 tablespoon chopped fresh basil, *or* ¼ teaspoon dried
   Freshly ground black pepper to taste
2 cloves garlic, peeled and mashed
1 small onion, diced
1 green pepper, diced
1 red pepper, diced
¼ pound mushrooms, sliced

In a medium saucepan, boil some water. Drop the tomatoes in the boiling water for 30 seconds each; then remove with tongs. Peel them and chop loosely.

Melt the margarine in a skillet over medium heat. Add the tomatoes, oregano, basil, and black pepper, and sauté until tender, about 10 minutes. Add the garlic, onion, and peppers, and simmer for about 15 minutes. Then add the mushrooms and simmer an additional 5–10 minutes.

While the sauce is cooking, bring the 4 quarts water to a boil and add the pasta. Cook according to package instructions or as long as you like (10 minutes is usually plenty for most kinds of pasta; if you love yours truly al dente, cook it less).

When done, drain and rinse pasta with warm water, and put in a bowl. Pour the sauce over the drained pasta and serve. SERVES 2–4, depending on how much pasta you make.

Spaghetti alla Marinara

        Spaghetti, as much as you need
    4 quarts water

    SAUCE:
    2 onions, chopped
    2 tablespoons chicken stock, *or* 2 low-sodium bouillon
        cubes melted in ¼ cup water
    1 tablespoon finely chopped fresh rosemary, *or* 1
        teaspooon dried
    2 cloves garlic, crushed
    2 14-ounce cans tomatoes, drained
    ¼ cup tomato sauce
        Dash salt
        Freshly ground black pepper to taste
    ½ teaspoon sugar
    2 cups sliced mushrooms

Cook the onions in the stock until soft. Add the rosemary and garlic, and sauté gently for a minute longer. Stir in the tomatoes, tomato sauce, salt, pepper, and sugar. Simmer uncovered, for 10–15 minutes.

While sauce is simmering, cook spaghetti according to package instructions. When just a few minutes remain before the spaghetti is done, mix the mushrooms in the sauce and stir. Return sauce to a boil, lower heat, and simmer for 3 minutes.

When spaghetti is done, drain, rinse with warm water, and put into a serving bowl. Pour sauce over it, and serve immediately.
SERVES 2–4, depending on the amount of pasta you made.

Spaghetti with Asparagus

This delicious meal takes only about 15 minutes to prepare. The only trick lies in having the pasta and the asparagus finish cooking at about the same time. Follow the instructions carefully, and the meal is easy to pull off.

> Spaghetti for 2–4 people (½–1 pound altogether)
> 4 quarts water
> ½ pound thin asparagus, tough ends discarded and
>   the stalks sliced into 1-inch pieces
> 2 tablespoons unsalted margarine or butter
> Pinch white pepper
> ¼ cup grated Parmesan cheese

Put the water on to boil, so that it will be ready when it's time to add the spaghetti.

Next, in a skillet over medium heat, melt the margarine or butter. Add the asparagus to the skillet and sauté for about 5 minutes.

By now the water should be boiling (if it's not, remove the asparagus from the heat until it is). Add the spaghetti and cook for about 5 minutes, or until it is as you like it.

After you have added the pasta to the boiling water, add the pepper to the asparagus and cook for 3–5 minutes longer.

When the pasta is done, drain, rinse with cold water, and put in a serving dish. Pour the asparagus over it, toss with the cheese, and serve.

SERVES 2–4

RICE

Curried Spinach Rice

> ¼ cup water
> 1 small onion, chopped
> 1 cup cooked chopped spinach (frozen is fine)
> ½ teaspoon low-sodium soy sauce
> ½ teaspoon curry powder
> ½ teaspoon ground coriander
> 1½ cups cooked long-grain brown rice
> 1 ripe tomato, sliced
> ¼ cup blanched almonds

Preheat oven to 350°.

In a large skillet, bring the water to a boil. Add the onion and stirfry over medium heat until softened. Add the spinach, cover, and steam over low heat until tender, about 5–10 minutes (check to make sure there's enough water so the spinach doesn't burn). Add the soy sauce, curry, coriander, and rice, mix well, and remove from heat.

Pour the mixture into a greased square baking dish. Layer the sliced tomatoes over the top. Bake for 25–30 minutes. When done, sprinkle the blanched almonds over the top and serve.
SERVES 3

Herbed Wild Rice with Brown Rice

3 cups low-sodium chicken stock (skim off fat if
   possible)
½ cup wild rice
½ cup long-grain brown rice
2 tablespoons minced scallions
2 cloves garlic, minced or crushed
1 teaspoon low-sodium soy sauce
½ teaspooon thyme
½ teaspoon dried chervil *or* chopped fresh parsley
½ teaspoon dried basil *or* 1 teaspoon fresh, chopped
2 bay leaves

In a medium saucepan, bring ¼ cup of the stock to a boil. Add
the wild rice, rice, scallions, garlic, and soy sauce and stirfry
for 2–3 minutes until the vegetables are soft. Now put the
remaining stock and seasonings in the pan and bring to a boil.

Reduce heat to low, and cook for 1 hour or until the rice is
tender. Take out the bay leaves and continue to cook, uncovered, until all the liquid has evaporated.
SERVES 4–6

Orange-flavored Rice

1 cup brown rice
1 cup cold water
2 teaspoons orange juice
1 teaspoon unsalted margarine

Combine rice, water, orange juice, and margarine in a sauce-pan, and place over high heat until water starts to boil. Stir once with a fork. Reduce heat, cover, and simmer 15–20 minutes, or until liquid is absorbed. If the rice is not moist enough, stir in a little more orange juice and serve.

SERVES 4

VEGETABLES

Artichokes

8 medium artichokes, whole
1 teaspoon safflower oil
  Juice of 1 lemon
2 lemons, cut in half
1 clove garlic, whole
2 tablespoons chopped fresh basil
  Mustard Sauce (see page 184)

Cut the bottoms off the artichokes and with a scissors, cut off the sharp tips. It will take a little time, but if you've ever had an artichoke thorn in your finger, you know this is time well spent.

Take two of your largest pots and put 4 artichokes in each. Add about two inches of water and half the oil, lemon juice, lemon halves, garlic, and basil to each pot. Cook, covered, for about 45 minutes. (To check if the artichokes are ready, pull a leaf from each pot and taste.)

When done, remove the artichokes from the pots with tongs, draining any excess liquid. Place the artichokes on a platter and chill in the refrigerator.

Make the mustard sauce. Serve in individual dishes with each artichoke.
SERVES 8

Green Bean Guacamole

> 1 16-ounce package frozen green beans
> ½ cup nonfat plain yogurt
> ¼ cup canned green chile salsa
> ¼ cup chopped onions
> 2 tablespoons chopped celery
> 1 tablespoon onion powder
> ½ tablespoon finely chopped, seeded jalapeño chile
> 1 teaspoon dry mustard
> 1 teaspoon garlic powder
> 3 hard-boiled egg whites, chopped
> 1 tomato, chopped

Place the green beans in a steamer basket and set over boiling water in a saucepan. Cover and cook until all the beans are tender. Place the beans in a colander, and using a potato masher or the back of a large spoon, press out some of the liquid so that the beans are quite dry. Place the beans in a blender or food processor with all the other ingredients except the egg whites and tomato. Blend at moderate speed until the mixture is smooth. Now add the egg whites and tomato by hand. Chill before serving.
MAKES 2 CUPS

Note: You can serve this in a red cabbage that has been scooped out like a bowl, with homemade or no-salt potato chips, crackers, or raw vegetables, or as a topping for a salad. For a special snack, spread the guacamole on an oven-warmed corn tortilla, garnish as you would a taco, then roll or fold, and enjoy.

Carrots

Carrots are easy to make, delicious, and full of nutrients you can't do without. One cup of cooked carrots (fresh, not canned) has 51 grams of calcium, 340 milligrams of potassium, and get ready for this, 16,000 units of vitamin A (the FDA only requires 5,000 a day, so see how ahead of the game you can be?).

Generally, you don't have to peel carrots (there are vitamins in the skin). So forget what mom told you—you can cook them with the skin intact. Cooking them in about an inch of boiling water for 10 minutes should do it. Be sure to use a low flame because carrots burn easily.

VARIATIONS:
When the carrots are done, try the following as toppings:

1 tablespoon margarine, 1 tablespoon lemon juice, and a pinch of dried dill

1 tablespoon margarine and a pinch of cinnamon and/or cloves

1 tablespoon margarine, ¼ teaspoon dried basil, and 1 teaspoon parsley (or you can use parsley alone)

1 tablespoon margarine, a pinch of curry, and a pinch of ginger

1 tablespoon honey and/or 1 tablespoon unsweetened orange jam

Carrots in Lemon Cups

4 pounds carrots, washed well but not peeled
1 cup plain nonfat yogurt
1 cup chopped scallions
1 tablespoon chopped fresh dill
6 large lemons

Steam the carrots until they're tender. Blend in your food processor until smooth. Add yogurt and blend again. (You can season to taste with a pinch of salt if you must.) Put the carrot mixture in a bowl, add the scallions and dill, and mix gently.

Cut the lemons in half, and squeeze on a juicer so the halves stay nice and round (save lemon juice for some other use). Slice just the tip of the lemon half so it will stand as a cup. Now fill each half with the carrot purée and serve.
SERVES 12

Note: If you want to get really fancy, you can put the carrot mixture in a pastry bag and squeeze it out into a pattern in the lemon halves.

Carrots in Orange Juice

4 carrots
⅓ cup orange juice
¾ cup water
   Pinch salt
1 tablespoon honey or raw sugar
1 teaspoon fresh or dried dill
   Lemon slices (optional)

Wash the carrots, and slice in your food procesor or by hand (make sure the "coins" are thin).

Put the carrots in a small pot; add the orange juice, water, salt, and honey, and cook, covered, over low heat for about an hour. Check every now and then to make sure all the liquid has not evaporated. If it has, add a little more water or juice.

When done, put on a serving platter, garnish with the dill (you can also add lemon slices), and serve. This dish is also good cold.
SERVES 2–4

Cauliflower

Another vegetable goodie—mother wasn't kidding when she said that vegetables were good for you. Listen to this—1 cup cooked fresh cauliflower has 260 mgs of potassium and 69 mgs of vitamin C. Nothing to sneer at—we get it where we can!

The first step with cauliflower, according to most cauliflower addicts, is to cut the head into buds and soak them in water. Then put the buds into a steamer and cook for 10–15 minutes. My best friend adds lemon juice to the cauliflower while it is cooking, and at the last minute, adds tarragon (the taste of tarragon is consistent with the lemon juice—both are tart).

VARIATIONS:
Toppings for cauliflower:

1 tablespoon margarine and a pinch of dill

1 tablespoon margarine and 2 tablespoons chopped, fresh basil

1 tablespoon margarine and 1 teaspoon grated Parmesan cheese

Or saute an equal amount of halved Brussels sprouts with the cauliflower in one teaspoon margarine until brown

Corn

A word about corn—I have always preferred eating fresh corn on the cob, because it is delicious and because it is a good source of potassium and vitamin A. But in researching the contents of food, I found out that compared to fresh corn frozen corn has twice the amount of carbohydrates, 45% more phosphorus, and nearly double the amount of vitamin A.

Cook fresh or frozen corn in boiling water for 7–10 minutes. Drain and, to frozen corn, add 1 tablespoon margarine and any of the following seasonings: parsley, chopped onions, garlic powder, curry powder, or 1 tablespoon plain nonfat yogurt.

Eggplant–Tomato Stew

　　　1 large eggplant, peeled and diced
　　　1 large green pepper, chopped
　　　1 large onion, chopped
　　　4 cloves garlic, minced or crushed
　　　1 cup vegetable stock or water
　　　1 16-ounce can diced (or crushed) tomatoes, with
　　　　　juice
　　　¼ cup canned low-sodium tomato paste
　　　1 15-ounce can pinto beans, drained
　　1½ teaspoons low-sodium soy sauce
　　1½ teaspoons chili powder
　　　1 teaspoon garlic powder
　　　1 teaspoon onion powder
　　　1 teaspoon curry powder
　　　1 teaspoon ground cumin

Place the eggplant, green pepper, onion, garlic, and ¼ cup of the stock or water in a large pot. Bring to a boil, reduce to medium heat, and sauté the vegetables for 10 minutes, stirring constantly. You want the liquid to evaporate, but be sure the vegetables don't burn.

Now add the remaining stock or water and all the other ingredients, stir well, and return to a boil. Reduce the heat to low and cook, covered, for 25 minutes. Serve.
MAKES ABOUT 6 CUPS

Note: If you want, you can keep a supply of this dish in your refrigerator. It keeps well up to 3 days.

Gazpacho Mold

> 1 cup canned (low-sodium) tomato or V-8 juice
> 1 envelope plus 1 teaspoon unflavored gelatin
> ½ tablespoon red wine vinegar
>   Dash Tabasco
> ¾ cup peeled and diced tomatoes
> ½ cup peeled, seeded, and chopped cucumber
> ½ cup diced carrots
> ¼ cup chopped green pepper
> ⅛ cup finely chopped red onion
> ⅛ cup finely chopped scallions or chives
> 1½ tablespoons canned green chile salsa
>   Watercress or parsley sprigs for garnish

Place ¾ cup of the tomato juice in a saucepan and add the gelatin. Let soak briefly, then set the saucepan over low heat and stir constantly until the gelatin is dissolved.

Remove from the heat and stir in the remaining tomato juice, vinegar, and Tabasco. Chill to the consistency of unbeaten egg white.

When chilled, fold in the chopped vegetables and salsa, combining well. Pour the mixture into a 1½-quart mold and chill until firm. Unmold and garnish with watercress or parsley sprigs.
SERVES 4–6

Stuffed Mushrooms

       30 large mushrooms
        1 large (1 pound) eggplant
       ¼ cup chopped scallions
          Pinch salt
          Freshly ground black pepper to taste
        1 teaspoon dried basil
       ¼ teaspoon Tabasco
       ½ cup lemon juice
        1 cup water
       ½ cup grated Parmesan cheese
          Parsley sprigs for garnish

Preheat oven to 400°.

Make several cuts in the eggplant; put in a glass casserole and bake for 30–40 minutes or until soft. Remove from the oven, cool, and skin. Cut the eggplant into small pieces. Mix with the scallions, salt, pepper, basil, and Tabasco, and then blend in the food processor for about 30 seconds.

Clean the mushrooms with a mushroom brush. Remove and discard stems; wash caps well, and dry. In a pot, boil the lemon juice and water, and add the mushroom caps. Cook for about a minute. Drain and place, bottom sides up, in a greased casserole.

Fill each mushroom cap with the eggplant mixture, leaving a little room at the top. Sprinkle with the Parmesan cheese. Bake for about 15 minutes. Serve on a large platter garnished with parsley.
SERVES 18

Sherried Mushrooms

½ pound fresh mushrooms, sliced
½ tablespoon unsalted margarine
2 tablespoons dry sherry
Freshly ground black pepper to taste

In a skillet over medium heat, sauté mushrooms in margarine for 5 minutes. Add sherry and toss. Sauté until all the liquid disappears. Transfer to serving dish, season with pepper, and serve.
SERVES 3

Potato–Vegetable Casserole

   4 ounces Parmesan cheese, shredded
   ¾ cup nonfat plain yogurt
   1 teaspoon Dijon mustard
     Freshly ground black pepper to taste
   3 potatoes, boiled, peeled, and thinly sliced
   1 cup cauliflower florets, steamed
   1 cup thinly sliced carrots, steamed
   ¼ cup chopped scallions

Preheat broiler.

In a small bowl, combine the first four ingredients. In a shallow 2-quart casserole, arrange potatoes, cauliflower, and carrots. Sprinkle with scallions and top with yogurt mixture. Broil until cheese is melted and begins to brown, about 7 minutes. Serve immediately.
SERVES 2

Stuffed Baked Potatoes

   2 baking potatoes
   1 tablespoon unsalted margarine
   4 tablespoons milk
     Freshly ground black pepper to taste

Bake potatoes in a 450° oven for 45–60 minutes. Remove from the oven and cut in half lengthwise. Scoop out the contents with a teaspoon. Reserve skins. Mash insides by hand or in your food processor (use quick on-and-off strokes so the po-

tatoes don't get sticky), add margarine, milk, and pepper. Then spoon mashed potato into the shells. Bake for 15 minutes, then serve.
SERVES 4

VARIATIONS:
Top the potatoes with one of the following:

½ tablespoon grated Parmesan cheese

1 teaspoon grated onion, sautéed

1 teaspoon chopped chives

2 mushrooms cut in pieces and sautéed

½ teaspoon curry powder

½ teaspoon nutmeg

1 tablespoon nonfat plain yogurt, 1 teaspoon chives, and 1 teaspoon grated onion

2 tablespoons nonfat plain yogurt and a pinch of dill

Baked Sweet Potatoes

Wash and dry as many medium sweet potatoes as you need. Bake in a 450° oven until tender, about 30 minutes. (If you want the skin to be soft, rub a little unsalted margarine on it before baking.)

VARIATIONS:
Slice open the top of each potato and spoon in any of the following:

1 tablespoon low-sodium peanut butter

1 tablespoon unsalted margarine, mixed with a pinch of nutmeg and, if you wish, ¼ teaspoon sherry or Cointreau

1 tablespoon honey mixed with 1 tablespoon melted unsalted margarine

Yam Bowls

    4 oranges
    1 16-ounce can yams
    1 tablespoon unsalted margarine
    1 tablespoon flaked coconut, for garnish

Preheat oven to 350°.

Cut the oranges in half and squeeze gently, saving the juice. Carefully scoop out the rest of the orange, leaving a clean shell.

In a blender or food processor, blend the yams with the orange juice and margarine until they are creamy smooth.

If you have a pastry bag, fill it with the yam mixture and then fill each orange half. If you don't have one, merely spoon the yam mixture into each orange half.

Put the oranges in a glass casserole and bake for 20 minutes. Garnish with the coconut, and serve.
SERVES 4 (You can make this for as many people as you like; figure 1–2 halves per person.)

Ratatouille

> 1 eggplant, peeled and cubed
> 1 small onion, sliced
> ½ cup chicken stock
> 1 clove garlic, crushed
> 2 green peppers, seeded and diced
> 4 ripe tomatoes, peeled and chopped
> ½ teaspoon dried thyme
> 1 teaspoon dried oregano
> Freshly ground black pepper to taste
> Chopped parsley, for garnish

Rinse the cubed eggplant in a colander, and let drain for 20–30 minutes. Rinse again and pat dry.

In a stockpot over medium heat, cook the onion in the stock, and then add the garlic, peppers, and tomatoes as you finish preparing them. Add the eggplant, thyme, oregano, and black pepper. Reduce heat, cover, and cook gently for another 20–30 minutes, stirring from time to time. If there is too much liquid when done, drain.

Sprinkle with chopped parsley. Serve hot, or cold on a bed of lettuce leaves.
SERVES 2–3

Sautéed Cherry Tomatoes

> ½ pound cherry tomatoes
> ½ tablespoon unsalted margarine
> 1 clove garlic, crushed
> 2 tablespoons chopped fresh basil, *or* ¾ teaspoon dried

Wash the tomatoes and dry well. Melt the margarine in a skillet over medium heat. Add garlic and sauté for 30 seconds (don't burn it!). Add tomatoes and sauté quickly, constantly shaking pan and tossing tomatoes, making sure not to break skins. Now add the basil and sauté another minute.

This is wonderful as a side dish with fish or as a sauce poured over plain pasta.
SERVES 2–3

Zucchini with Herbs and Tomatoes

>2 medium zucchini
>1 tablespoon unsalted margarine
>1 drop olive oil
>1 small onion, chopped
>1 clove garlic, minced
>1 bay leaf
>1 teaspoon basil
>½ teaspoon oregano
>   Freshly ground black pepper to taste
>1 teaspoon raw sugar
>1 tomato, peeled and cut up

Wash the zucchini (but don't peel them—there are vitamins in them there skins!), and cut into thin "coins."

Stir the margarine and oil together in a frying pan over medium heat, add the onion and garlic, and cook for 5–7 minutes (but don't brown). Add the zucchini, herbs, and pepper. Stir, and add a little water to moisten. Cover, and cook 10 minutes. Then add the sugar and tomato and cook until tender, about 5–7 minutes.
SERVES 2–3

BREADS AND MUFFINS

Berry Bran Muffins

1 cup unprocessed bran
⅔ cup whole wheat flour
⅔ cup white flour
1½ teaspoons baking soda
1 egg
¼ cup oil
⅓ cup honey
1½ cups nonfat plain yogurt
1 cup frozen berries (any that you like), thawed and
  drained

Preheat oven to 400°.

Grease a 12-cup muffin pan with margarine. In a bowl, gently mix the bran, flours, and baking soda. In another bowl, beat the egg, oil, and honey until well blended.

In a blender or food processor, blend the yogurt until it is smooth. Add the yogurt and the bran mixture to the egg mixture and stir them all together. Now gently stir in the berries.

Fill the muffin cups about ¾ full with the batter. Bake for 20–25 minutes, checking to make sure they don't burn. They are done when they are lightly browned.
MAKES 12 MUFFINS

Note: If you have extra muffins left over, simply wrap them individually in freezer wrap and store in the freezer. When you want one, unwrap it and warm for 10 minutes in your oven or toaster oven.

Spiced Zucchini Muffins

 1 cup unprocessed bran
 ⅔ cup whole wheat flour
 ⅔ cup flour
 2 teaspoons baking soda
 1 egg
 ¼ cup oil
 ⅓ cup brown sugar
 1 teaspoon ground cinnamon
 ¼ teaspoon ground cloves
 1 teaspoon ground orange peel (sold in the spice
    section at the market)
 1 cup nonfat milk
 1 cup zucchini, unpeeled and grated
 ½ cup chopped nuts

Preheat oven to 400°.

Grease a 12-cup muffin pan with margarine. In a bowl, mix together the bran, the flours, and the baking soda.

In another bowl, blend the egg, oil, sugar, spices, and orange peel until they are thoroughly mixed. Then add the milk and zucchini, mix well, and stir in the nuts.

Fill each muffin cup about ¾ full with the batter. Bake for 30 minutes. Then remove from the pan and let cool.
MAKES 12

Note: Individually wrap any leftover muffins you don't eat and freeze them. When you want one, unwrap it and warm for 10 minutes in your oven or toaster oven.

Popovers

I've had a love affair with popovers for years but until recently believed that I could only satisfy my cravings in restaurants. Now, thanks to one of my girlfriends, I have learned how to make them at home. It is so easy that I can make them for breakfast while I am getting ready to go to work on the set.

>   2 eggs
>   1 cup nonfat milk
>   1 cup sifted flour
>   ½ teaspoon salt

Preheat oven to 375°.

Lightly beat the eggs. Add the milk, sifted flour, and salt. Mix lightly and disregard the lumps.

Grease a 6-cup muffin pan or a popover pan (the latter are usually made of cast iron and are deeper than muffin pans). Fill each cup about ¾ full and place pan in the oven. (If you are only making 4 popovers and the pan is made for 6, fill the two empty cups ¾ full of water.) Turn your oven to 450°. Bake for 20 minutes. Remove and eat immediately.

MAKES 6–8 popovers in a muffin pan, 4–6 in a popover pan.

DESSERTS

Apple Pie (That's Good for You)

Ready-made crust for a 9-inch pie
4 cups thinly sliced, peeled, cored apples, very green
   and sour
2 tablespoons lemon juice
½ cup raw sugar
½ teaspoon cinnamon
¼ teaspoon ground cloves
1 teaspoon vanilla
1 cup granola
¼ cup raisins (*or* 1 1½-ounce box)
1 tablespoon unsalted margarine

Preheat oven to 400°.

In a glass mixing bowl, mix the sliced apples with the lemon juice, sugar, cinnamon, cloves, vanilla, granola, and raisins.

Fill the unbaked pie shell with the apple mixture. (You can take the ready-made pie shell and put it in your own pretty pie dish—just gently push the dough to fit the dish.) Dot the top with the margarine.

Place the pie in the oven and bake for 15 minutes. Then lower the oven temperature to 350° and bake for another 20–25 minutes. Remove the pie from the oven and let cool.

Note: Sometimes, for vanity, I make a lattice topping for the pie. Ready-made crusts come two to a pack. I use one for the pie and take the other, re-roll it (adding a little flour), cut it into 7"–8" strips, and make a crisscross pattern on top of the pie.

Apple Rings in Sherry

    6 tart green apples
    2 tablespoons unsalted margarine
    2 tablespoons lemon juice
    ¼ teaspoon cinnamon
    ½ cup dry sherry
    ¼ cup brown sugar
    ¼ cup slivered almonds

Preheat broiler.

Core the apples but don't peel them. With a sharp knife, carefully slice them into ¼-inch rings.

Grease a glass baking dish. Arrange the apples in layers until they are all used up. Dot the top with the margarine, add the lemon juice, and sprinkle on the cinnamon. Pour the sherry over the apples, and sprinkle the top with the brown sugar.

Put the apples in the broiler until the sugar on top is melted, about 8–10 minutes. Sprinkle with the almonds, and return to the broiler for another minute. Serve warm.
SERVES 4–6

Honey Apples

This dessert is delicious, will satisfy your hunger for sweets, and is even good for you.

    4 medium cooking apples
    1 tablespoon chopped nuts, toasted
    1 tablespoon chopped dates
      Juice of ½ lemon
    2 tablespoons clear honey
    ½ teaspoon ground cinnamon

Preheat oven to 350°.

Wash and core the apples, and peel the top half. Place in an ovenproof dish (I use a small, porcelain soufflé dish). Mix the remaining ingredients together and fill the centers of the apples. Pour any leftover mixture over the apples and cook, covered with aluminum foil, in the oven for about 45 minutes. Serve warm.

SERVES 4

Banana–Berry Dessert

> 2 cups frozen unsweetened berries (use your favorite
> —strawberries, blueberries, boysenberries,
> raspberries, blackberries, etc.)
> ½ teaspoon liquid artificial sweetener
> 3 bananas
> 2 tablespoons cognac or brandy
> ¼ cup unsweetened orange juice
> 2 tablespoons chopped walnuts or slivered almonds,
> optional

Preheat oven to 350°.

Put the berries, frozen, in your blender or food processor, add the sweetener, and blend until smooth.

Slice the bananas diagonally, put in a saucepan, cover with the cognac and orange juice and sauté for about 3 minutes.

Now put the bananas in a glass baking dish and pour the berry sauce over them. Put in the oven and bake for 10 minutes.

When done, take out and place on a serving dish. If you like, you can garnish with the walnuts or almonds, and serve. I promise—you'll never miss the whipped cream.

SERVES 4–6

Honeydew Squash

Chill two champagne glasses. In your blender, combine 1 cup very ripe honeydew chunks and ½ cup chilled orange juice (no sugar added) and process until smooth. Now divide the mixture into chilled glasses and garnish each with a lemon slice. Serve immediately.
SERVES 2 (about ½ cup each)

FOR ADDITIONAL SERVINGS USE:

	3 servings	*4 servings*	*5 servings*
Honeydew	1½ cups	2 cups	3 cups
Orange juice	¾ cup	1 cup	1½ cups
Lemon slices	3	4	5

Mandarin Orange Soufflé

    5 oranges
    2 tablespoons Cointreau
    2 egg yolks (just this once!)
    1 tablespoon liquid artificial sweetener
    2 tablespoons flour
    ½ cup nonfat milk, warmed
    ½ cup orange juice
    ¼ cup lemon juice
    1 12-ounce can mandarin oranges
    3 egg whites

Preheat oven to 325°.

Grate the zest of one of the oranges and put in a small pan. Add the Cointreau and reduce over a low flame until all the liquid has disappeared. (Be careful not to burn—you must watch the pan at all times!) Set aside.

Cut the tops off the other oranges, and scoop out and discard the insides. (This is best done with a serrated curved knife, sometimes called a grapefruit knife.)

Combine the egg yolks with ½ tablespoon of the sweetener, and beat until the mixture turns light yellow, the color of a lemon. Slowly add the flour and the milk. Put it all in a small pan and cook over low heat, stirring constantly, until the mixture thickens. Put the mixture back in the bowl, and beat in the orange juice. Put it all back in the pot and cook again until it thickens. Set this custard aside to cool.

When cooled, add the orange zest and lemon juice. Drain the can of mandarin oranges, and put an equal amount in each of the scooped-out oranges. Do the same thing with most of the custard you made, leaving about a third. Beat the egg whites until stiff with the remaining ½ tablespoon of sweetener. Fold the extra custard into the egg whites and put a little bit into each of the oranges.

Take all the oranges and put into a glass casserole. Put water in the bottom, about 1 inch deep. Put into the oven and bake for 20 minutes. Let cool for a few minutes, and serve.
SERVES 4

Note: I usually do everything up until beating the egg whites while I am making dinner. Then I can do the rest later—otherwise, this is a lot to do at the end of an evening.

Pears in Rum

    4 pears
¼ cup lime juice
¼ cup honey
¾ cup rum
¼ cup water
  2 tablespoons chopped almonds for garnish

Preheat oven to 325°.

Peel and cut the pears in half, and core them. Arrange them cut side up in a glass baking dish.

In a small bowl, mix the lime juice, honey, and rum. Put 1 tablespoon of this mixture in the little hollow in each pear. You should have a small amount of the mixture left over.

Bake for 1 hour. While the pears are baking, mix the remaining juice mixture with the water and occasionally baste the pears with it.

When done, turn the pears over gently, sprinkle with the chopped almonds, and brown under the broiler for 3–4 minutes (if the nuts start burning, you've left the pears in too long!).

Remove pears from the broiler and transfer to individual bowls. Drizzle the remaining pan-juices over them, and serve. SERVES 4–8, depending on how many pear halves your guests can eat.

Note: If you like you can serve some yogurt, blended with a teaspoon of vanilla in the food processor, over the pears.

Sherbet Meringues

    1 package frozen raspberries
    ½ teaspoon vanilla
    3 pints lemon sherbet
    12 meringue pie shells (you can buy these in the
         market; you can also use 24 meringue cookies)
    12 fresh raspberries for garnish

Take 12 of your prettiest flat salad plates. Put them in the refrigerator for half an hour or more.

Put the frozen raspberries and the vanilla in your food processor and blend until very smooth.

Spread the 12 plates out on the counter. Place a meringue shell in the center of each plate. If you're using meringue cookies, place two on the side of each plate.

Now you have to hurry or the sherbet will melt before you finish serving. Take a scoop of the lemon sherbet and place it on each meringue shell or next to the cookies. Spoon on raspberry sauce and put a raspberry on top of the sherbet and serve quickly.

SERVES 12 (Obviously you can make as many or as few of these as you need for a dinner party.)

Quick Fruit Glaze

Heat ½ cup currant jelly until it melts. Spoon over fruit.

Use over peaches, for dessert, or as a sauce for cold meats (a great idea for plain, broiled, or baked veal!).

EXTRAS

Good-for-You-French Toast

    2 slices low-sodium bread
    1 egg, beaten
    ⅛ cup low-fat or nonfat milk
    ¼ cup raw sugar
    ½ teaspoon vanilla
    Nutmeg
    Honey, jelly, or plain nonfat yogurt for topping

Preheat your oven to 450°.

Remove crusts from bread slices. Mix together the egg, milk, sugar, and vanilla. Soak bread in mixture for 2 minutes, then flip over and soak an additional 2 minutes. Place slices on an oiled baking dish (don't overdo it—just a little oil, margarine, or Pam will do) or a nonstick pan.

Bake for 7 minutes on one side, then turn and brown 5 minutes longer. Sprinkle with nutmeg. Serve with honey, jelly, or plain nonfat yogurt.
MAKES 2 SLICES

Banana Yogurt Breakfast

    1 cup nonfat plain yogurt
    1 banana, sliced
    2 tablespoons chopped walnuts

Mix together and enjoy!

Hermien's Perfect Peanut Butter

Nutritionist Hermien Lee processes her own peanut butter to eliminate virtually all the oil in it. The result is a "candy" you can carry around with you for instant protein, and a spread you can use for breads or for recipes.

First buy old-fashioned peanut butter right in your supermarket. Pour off the oil. Now take a paper towel, place it at the top of the jar, close the lid, and turn the jar upside down. Place the jar on your counter and leave it there for about 15 minutes.

Now look at the jar—the paper towel will be saturated with oil (imagine that oil flowing through your body!). Remove that paper towel, throw it away, and put another one in. Again turn the jar upside down and wait for the towel to get saturated. Repeat this one more time (that's three times altogether).

Now open the jar, and with a knife make a funnel in the peanut butter. Roll one paper towel and push it into this funnel. Cover the jar with the lid and put it back on the counter. In about 24 hours, all the leftover oil will have been drawn into this paper towel.

What's left is "peanut candy," actually a hard concentration of peanut butter with absolutely no oil in it, and all the protein you want and need.

For a snack, take a teaspoon of the peanut butter and wrap it in foil. You can carry it around and eat it whenever you feel the need for some energy. Compare this to a chocolate bar with all its sugar and fat and you'll see what a wonderful and nutritious snack this is.

If you want to use it as peanut butter spread, just add a little water to a teaspoonful, or put a teaspoon of the candy on foil and heat in your toaster oven for 3 minutes.

Potato Chips

I first tasted these at a friend's and couldn't believe they had no salt or fat.

>   4 baking potatoes
>   4 cups of ice cold water

Preheat oven to 425°.

Slice the potatoes in your food processor so they come out in very thin slices. Put the slices in the ice water and leave them for about half an hour (the water will prevent the potatoes from turning brown).

Drain, and pat them all dry with paper towels.

Spread enough chips on a nonstick cookie sheet to fill the pan, making sure none of the chips overlap. Bake in the oven for about 5 minutes; when they get brown on one side, turn them over with tongs. Bake for another 5 minutes. Take out and let cool on a plate, and repeat the procedure until all the chips have been baked.

Taste one—now aren't you surprised at how good they are?

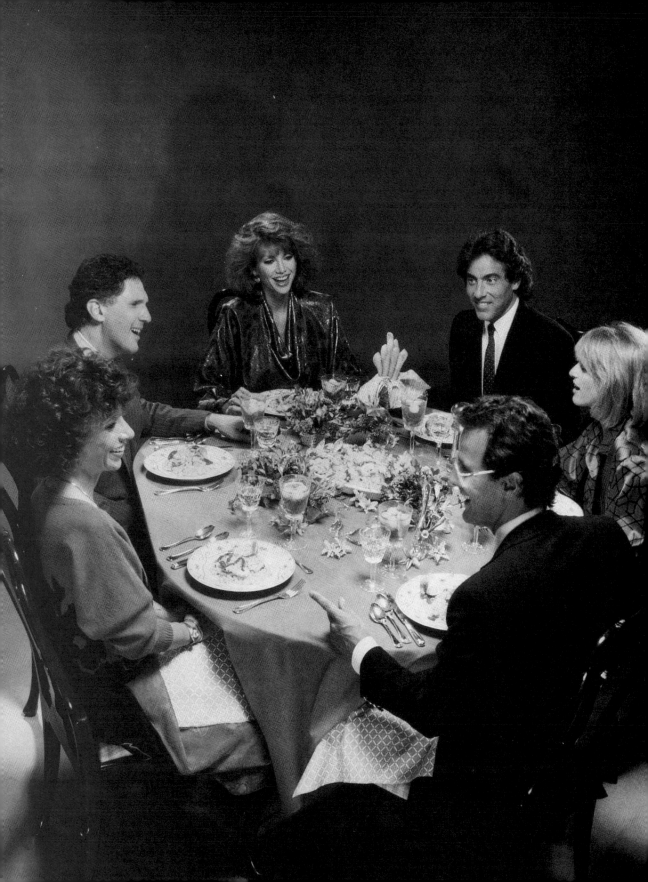

CHAPTER 5

ENTERTAINING AT HOME AND EATING OUT

I love a party, especially if I'm giving it. And why not? I love to bring out all the candles and place them nearly everywhere; I anticipate the sound of music rocking the room; I enjoy strewing colorful flowers in every corner; I relish planning the decor and choosing the dishes and coordinating the tablecloths and napkins; I like nothing more than sharing my home with my good friends (who also love a party!).

And, oh yes—the food. I love the food. I like to plan it, to cook it, and to eat it. I take especially great pleasure in watching my friends wolf down dishes I know they think are sinful. Salmon Mousse—Coffee Smoothies—Baked Rum Bananas—Shrimp and Orange Salad—Cioppino—Veal Stew—Yam Bowls—Chicken Vera Cruz—they disappear into the tummies of many who usually swear by creamed avocado soup, followed by steak smothered in bacon, finishing with fried bananas dipped in chocolate sauce. My dear friends and treasured guests never realize that I care about what they eat just as I care about what I eat, and that I serve them dishes that are not only beautiful and delicious but, perish the thought, actually good for them—foods that are as nutritious as possible.

I have always cooked for my guests just as I cook for myself and my own family, because I feel that by serving them the best foods, made with the freshest and most nutritious ingredients, I am giving them a gift. I don't eat fatty foods—why would I serve them to my guests? It seems to me that the premise of entertaining is caring for your guests, and that means not only providing them with candlelight, beautiful flowers, and good music but also serving food that shows just as much thoughtfulness, love, and concern.

It is easy to be on the Diet to Lose or the Diet for Life and entertain comfortably and successfully. Both diets are flexible enough for you to party without looking over your shoulder or feeling guilty about eating to your heart's content. The recipes I have used over the years are pleasing to the eye, delicious, and full of nutritious ingredients. And no one has ever noticed that they contain no salt, very little (if any) fat, and lots of the vitamins and minerals we all need.

I have never felt that I was shortchanging my friends by leaving out the fats and salt—I'm only shortchanging them on bad food. And the test of it is that more often than not, at the end of a party, whether it is a sit-down dinner for eight or a buffet for thirty I end up with several requests to share my recipes.

In addition to the more than one hundred recipes in the Diet for Life, many of which can be expanded for larger parties, I have compiled a list of recipes used for parties I have given over the years. All of these dishes can be eaten while on the Diet for Life (although some of them can be eaten on the Diet to Lose, I try to keep my partying down to a minimum while I am trying to lose weight).

I have put together six sample parties which contain both new recipes and some from the Diet for Life. These menus are

MENU

Dinner for Eight

Fruit Nectar Frappes

Veal Stew (p. 176)

Brown Rice

Steamed Vegetables with Parmesan (p. 107)

Green Salad with French Dressing (p. 238)

Cherries in Port

Decaffeinated Coffee or Hot Tea

Fruit Nectar Frappes

> 8 ounces each of pear, apricot, raspberry, and
>   strawberry nectars, and of papaya, tangerine, and
>   pink grapefruit juices
> ½ cup rum
> 1 cup nonfat plain yogurt
>   Mint leaves and/or fresh strawberries for garnish

In a bowl, mix the juices and nectars with the rum. Freeze overnight in ice cube trays. In the morning, take the frozen ice cubes and put them in your food processor. Chop the cubes, using steel blades. Add the yogurt, mix for another 30 seconds, then pour into chilled champagne or daiquiri glasses. Garnish with mint leaves and/or a strawberry in each glass.
SERVES 10–12

Cherries in Port

4 8-ounce cans sour Bing cherries, pitted
1 cup port wine

Pour all the cherries in a bowl. Take one cup of juice out and discard. Pour in the port wine, chill overnight. Serve in mini-bowls, with a cookie on the side.
SERVES 12

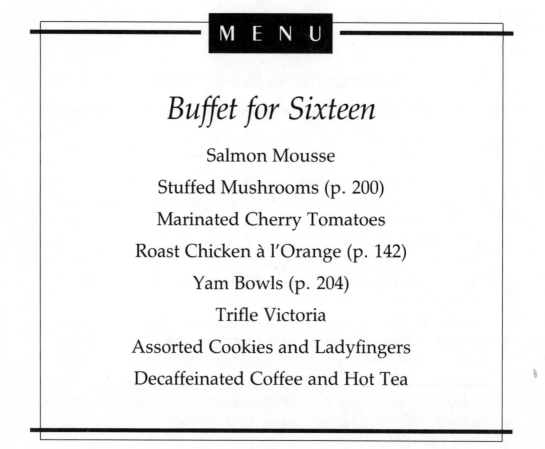

MENU

Buffet for Sixteen

Salmon Mousse

Stuffed Mushrooms (p. 200)

Marinated Cherry Tomatoes

Roast Chicken à l'Orange (p. 142)

Yam Bowls (p. 204)

Trifle Victoria

Assorted Cookies and Ladyfingers

Decaffeinated Coffee and Hot Tea

Salmon Mousse

> 2 15½-ounce cans red salmon, drained (red is more
>   expensive than pink, but you need it for color)
> 1 envelope unflavored gelatin
> ¼ cup cold water
> ½ cup boiling water
> ½ cup nonfat plain yogurt
> 1 tablespoon lemon juice
> 1 tablespoon finely chopped onion
> ¼ teaspoon Tabasco
> ¼ teaspoon paprika
>   Pinch salt
> 1 tablespoon capers, chopped (optional)
> 2 egg whites
>   Lemon slices, parsley, and strawberries (if available)
>   for garnish
>
> 1 teaspoon oil
> 1 metal mold in the shape of a fish

In a large bowl, soften the gelatin in cold water and add the boiling water. Stir until the gelatin is dissolved. Cool for 10 minutes, but don't let it harden. Then add the yogurt, lemon juice, onion, Tabasco, paprika, and salt, and mix well. Chill in the refrigerator until the mixture has the consistency of unbeaten egg whites. Now stir in the salmon and capers.

In a separate bowl, whip the egg whites until they're almost hard, then fold them into the salmon mixture.

Put the oil on a paper towel, and use the towel to oil the inside of the mold. Pour the salmon mixture into the mold and chill until hard. When you're ready to serve, ummold and turn over on a flat platter. You can garnish the sides of the mousse with lemon slices, parsley, and strawberries.

SERVES 12–18 (I have served this at a dinner party for 24 as an hors d'oeuvre and at a party for 12 as a side dish. The number of servings depends on how big your portions are.)

Marinated Cherry Tomatoes

      40 cherry tomatoes
      ⅓ cup red wine vinegar
      ¼ cup chopped scallions
      ½ teaspoon dried basil
      ¼ teaspoon dried oregano
      ½ teaspoon garlic powder
         Freshly ground black pepper to taste
      ½ cup vegetable oil
      1 head of cabbage

In your blender or food processor, blend all the ingredients except the tomatoes and cabbage. Wash and dry the tomatoes and put them in a salad bowl. Pour the dressing over the tomatoes, cover with foil, and refrigerate overnight.

Just before your party, drain the tomatoes (you can reserve the leftover dressing for some other use). Now arrange them on the head of cabbage by placing a toothpick through each one and sticking it into the cabbage. Place the cabbage on a platter and set it on the buffet or appetizer table. I sometimes surround the cabbage with green apples—it creates an unusual and pretty effect.

Trifle Victoria

> 2 packages frozen strawberries
> 2 packages Junkit brand Strawberry Danish dessert, *or*
>   1 6-ounce jar raspberry jam mixed with 2 cups
>   nonfat vanilla yogurt
>   Approximately 2 cups orange juice
> 4 packages ladyfingers
> 3 packages vanilla pudding
> 1 package whole fresh strawberries, cleaned and
>   stemmed

Thaw the frozen strawberries. Drain the syrup, and put the berries in one bowl and the syrup in another.

If using the Danish dessert, combine it in a saucepan with the orange juice and the syrup from the strawberries instead of using water as called for in the directions on the box. Bring to a boil and cook for 1 minute. Add the thawed strawberries and set the pot aside to cool.

If using the jam and yogurt, mix together with the thawed strawberries and set aside.

Make the vanilla pudding as directed, and cool in a pan of cold water to keep a film from forming.

Line the bottom and sides of a large glass bowl (preferably with straight sides) with a layer of ladyfingers. Cover with a thin layer of vanilla pudding, then a thin layer of the strawberry mixture. Gently place successive layers of lady-fingers, pudding, and strawberry mixture, then another layer of lady-fingers, another of pudding, and a last, thick layer of the strawberry mixture. If you have any ladyfingers left, you can top with those. Arrange the fresh strawberries on top, and refrigerate until you're ready to serve.

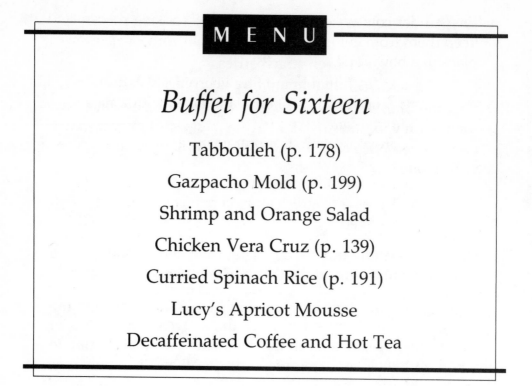

MENU

Buffet for Sixteen

Tabbouleh (p. 178)

Gazpacho Mold (p. 199)

Shrimp and Orange Salad

Chicken Vera Cruz (p. 139)

Curried Spinach Rice (p. 191)

Lucy's Apricot Mousse

Decaffeinated Coffee and Hot Tea

Shrimp and Orange Salad

        32 medium shrimp, peeled and deveined
        3 oranges
            Low-calorie, Low-sodium Vinaigrette Dressing
            (pg. 180)
        1 cup chopped fresh chives or scallions
        2 whole chives for garnish
        1 head butter or red leaf lettuce, or a mixture of the
            two

Throw the peeled shrimp into a pot of boiling water. Return
water to boil and simmer for 3–4 minutes. Drain shrimp and

rinse under cold water (this will stop the cooking process and keep them from getting chewy). Dry them with a paper towel, place in a bowl, and refrigerate.

Peel the oranges, making sure to remove all the white. Slice them with your cutting board over a bowl to catch the juice. If you like, you can chop the oranges—it will work just as well. Refrigerate.

In your food processor or blender, prepare the vinaigrette. While it's mixing, remove the shrimp and oranges from the refrigerator and mix together. Now pour the vinaigrette over the salad and return to the refrigerator until you're ready to serve. At the last minute mix in the chives or scallions. Serve on individual plates on a bed of lettuce, garnished with uncut chives.

Lucy's Apricot Mousse

> 1 8-ounce can apricots, drained, liquid reserved
> 1 package of lemon-flavored, artificially sweetened gelatin
> 2 tablespoons brandy
> 1 cup low-fat vanilla yogurt
> ½ teaspoon vanilla
> 1 cup crumbled vanilla wafers
> A few whole strawberries, raspberries, or mint leaves for garnish

Drain the apricots. Add enough water to the apricot juice to make 1¼ cups liquid. Put the liquid in a small saucepan and boil. Add the gelatin and stir until dissolved. Let cool.

Add the apricots and brandy to the gelatin mixture. Pour into a bowl and refrigerate until the mixture has the consistency of jelly.

When ready, remove the bowl from the refrigerator. With a hand mixer, beat the mixture slowly while adding the vanilla yogurt and vanilla.

Pour half of the mixture into a pretty square or round glass serving-bowl. Sprinkle on the wafer crumbs and then add the rest of the mixture on top. Refrigerate until firm. Serve in small dessert dishes. Garnish with a strawberry, a raspberry, or a mint leaf. If you like large portions, make two mousses.

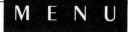

M E N U

Buffet for Twenty-four to Thirty

Assorted Bread Sticks and Crackers

Chick-pea Sesame Dip

Summer Rice Salad

Green Salad with French Dressing

Paella

Coffee Smoothies

Sunshine Orange Mold

Decaffeinated Coffee and Hot Tea

Chick-pea Sesame Dip

    1 cup commercially prepared sesame paste (tahini)
    2 cans chick-peas
    4 cloves garlic, peeled and mashed
    4 tablespoons lemon juice
    2 tablespoons olive oil (vegetable oil is also OK)

This is always a favorite dip for parties—it may be Middle Eastern in origin, but it has become a popular American dish, one which my guests relish. A word here about chick-peas. They are high in calories—1 cup has over 700! But since you don't eat one cup at a sitting, especially in this dip where two cups will serve at least 8–10 people, and since chick-peas have a large amount of potassium and calcium, this is both a delicious and nutritious dish.

First put all the ingredients in a food processor or blender and mix until you have a thick paste. Remove mixture to a small serving bowl. Garnish with slices of lemon and/or parsley leaves. Serve with pita bread (you can get this Middle Eastern bread in almost any supermarket) cut up into triangles. (You can also toast the pita triangles so they crunch like crackers, or serve any other crackers that you have on hand.)
SERVES 8–10

Summer Rice Salad

 2 cups brown rice, cooked and chilled (you can use
  white rice if you prefer)
 4 tomatoes, chopped
 2 tablespoons chopped fresh parsley
 ¼ cup chopped scallions
 ¼ cup sliced radishes, red or white
 ⅓ cup chopped celery
 ½ cup peeled and chopped cucumber
 ¼ cup oil
 1 tablespoon wine vinegar
 ¼ teaspoon prepared mustard
  Pinch paprika
  Pinch garlic powder
  Freshly ground black pepper to taste
  Pinch salt

In a bowl, combine the chilled rice with the tomatoes, parsley, scallions, radishes, celery, and cucumbers.

In your blender or food processor, mix the rest of the ingredients. Pour this dressing over the rice salad and mix. Chill in the refrigerator until ready to serve.
(This will keep in the refrigerator for 2–3 days.)

Note: Serving this salad in an attractive and interesting way has become a challenge for me. I like it in melon cups—I take a small melon and cut it in half, scoop out the seeds, and fill it with the salad. The combination of the sweet and sour tastes is very good. I have also served it on lettuce, in red cabbage leaves, and in papaya halves.

Green Salad with French Dressing

    1 head butter (Boston) lettuce
    1 head radicchio lettuce
    1 bunch arugula
  ½ pound spinach, washed and dried well
    1 bunch scallions or chives, chopped
    4 tablespoons chopped fresh parsley
1½ pounds mushrooms, sliced

DRESSING:
  ½ cup olive or other vegetable oil
    1 teaspoon Dijon mustard
    2 cloves garlic, mashed
  ½ teaspoon dried basil
  ⅛ teaspoon pepper
    3 tablespoons red wine vinegar
    2 tablespoons lemon juice

Wash the lettuce, arugula, and spinach well, then tear into bite-sized pieces. Dry well; mix with the scallions or chives, the parsley, and the mushrooms, and refrigerate.

To make the dressing, combine all the ingredients and blend in your food processor or blender. Pour over the salad when ready to serve.

Paella

3 cups uncooked white rice
1 teaspoon saffron
3 pounds cooked shrimp
2 8-ounce packages frozen crab
3 cans minced clams, with liquid
2 pounds cooked crayfish (optional)
3 16-ounce cans whole Italian tomatoes
6 cloves garlic, mashed
2 green peppers, chopped
1 red pepper, chopped
6 cups shredded cooked chicken

Cook the rice in chicken broth instead of water. When the rice is done, add the saffron and mix lightly with a fork.

Put the rice into a large saucepan or skillet. Add all the other ingredients and cook over a low flame until everything is heated. When done, put into a large serving dish. You can keep the paella warm on a warming tray on a buffet (be sure to cover the dish with aluminum foil until you are ready to serve).

SERVES AT LEAST 24

Coffee Smoothies

4 cups lowfat vanilla yogurt
½ cup brown sugar
2 tablespoons instant espresso or coffee
1 teaspoon vanilla
½ cup slivered almonds
Chocolate mocha beans for garnish

In your food processor, cream the yogurt for 15 seconds. Add the brown sugar, coffee, and vanilla, and mix for another 15 seconds. Refrigerate the mixture for a couple of hours if possible.

About an hour before your party, pour the mixture into wine or champagne glasses. Sprinkle on top with nuts and one or two of the chocolate beans. Return to the refrigerator until you're ready to serve.
Make this twice for generous portions.

Sunshine Orange Mold

This is pretty, delicious, and not bad for you—what more could you ask for?

> 3½ cups apricot nectar
> 2 packages orange Jell-O
> ½ cup orange juice
> ¼ cup grated carrot
> 1 can mandarin oranges
> ¼ cup dates, pitted and finely chopped
> 3 oranges

> Fruit-shaped mold, lightly greased

The trick here is to make the Jell-O using fruit juices instead of water.

In a small saucepan, heat the apricot nectar. While it is heating, put the Jell-O powder in a bowl. When the juice is hot, pour 2 cups of it over the Jell-O and stir until all the powder is dissolved. Add the remaining 1½ cups of apricot nectar and the orange juice, carrot, mandarin oranges, and dates and mix again. Pour the whole thing into the mold and chill for a few hours, until set.

While the Jell-O is hardening, take the oranges and slice them about ⅛″ thin. Take a large platter and cover with layers of the sliced oranges. When the Jell-O is ready, unmold and place on the bed of oranges. For added color, I sometimes sprinkle an arrangement of assorted berries, depending on which are in season, around the mold.

SERVES 8–12 for a dessert at a sit down dinner, 24 at a buffet.

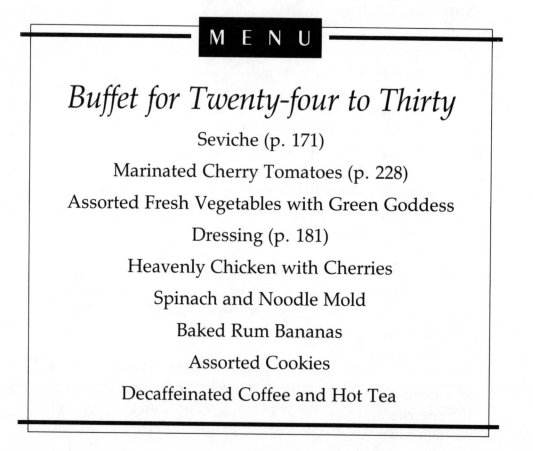

MENU

Buffet for Twenty-four to Thirty

Seviche (p. 171)

Marinated Cherry Tomatoes (p. 228)

Assorted Fresh Vegetables with Green Goddess

Dressing (p. 181)

Heavenly Chicken with Cherries

Spinach and Noodle Mold

Baked Rum Bananas

Assorted Cookies

Decaffeinated Coffee and Hot Tea

Heavenly Chicken with Cherries

This is one time I do *not* skin the chicken. It's too much work for a party, and it's too expensive to have the butcher do it. One time won't hurt!

       50 pieces chicken
        2 cups unsalted margarine, melted
        1 teaspoon finely ground black pepper
        3 cups water
        2 cups golden raisins
     1½ cups brown sugar
        8 cloves garlic, mashed
        5 onions, sliced thin
        1 bottle low-sodium chili sauce
        2 tablespoons low-sodium Worcestershire sauce
        3 16-ounce cans Bing cherries, pitted and drained
        2 cups sherry or port (whichever you prefer)

Preheat oven to "Broil."

You will probably need 3 roasting pans for this recipe. If you don't own that many, just buy the aluminum-foil disposable ones at any market.

Wash the chicken and dry well. Put the pieces in a single layer in each roasting pan, with the skin side up. Season with the pepper and broil for 15–20 minutes, until the skin is brown (you may want to turn it over halfway through to ensure browning on all sides).

In a large bowl, mix together all the other ingredients except the cherries and the sherry. Pour the mixture evenly over the chicken pieces and cover the pans with aluminum foil. Turn the oven down to 350° and bake the chicken for about an hour, basting as often as necessary to keep the meat moist.

When the meat is done, remove the aluminum foil, pour the cherries and sherry over the chicken, and bake, uncovered, in the oven for another 15 minutes.

When done, arrange the chicken on large platters, pour the sauce over the meat, and serve as soon as possible. This chicken can be kept warm on a warming tray (just keep it covered with the aluminum foil).
SERVES 24 (You can determine how many this recipe will serve by the number of chicken pieces you use. If you have extra sauce, freeze it and use it again at another time. If you need more sauce, add water and/or chicken broth to it.)

Spinach and Noodle Mold

> 3 packages flat noodles
> 6 packages frozen spinach, defrosted and drained
> ½ cup margarine
> 3 onions, chopped
> 4 eggs, lightly beaten
> 2 cups nonfat plain yogurt
> 3 molds in any attractive shape

Preheat oven to 350°.

In a large pot, bring 4 quarts of water to a boil. Cook the noodles (you may have to cook them in bunches, unless you have a huge pot) and drain. Put them into a large casserole and mix in the defrosted spinach.

In a saucepan, melt the margarine over medium heat and sauté the onions until lightly browned. Add the eggs and yogurt and mix with a wooden spoon.

Now grease the three molds with a little margarine. Pour the mixture into each mold until ¾ full.

Take three glass baking dishes, and fill each with water about half full. Put one mold in each casserole and put the casseroles in the oven (use two shelves or two separate ovens, if you have them). Bake for about 50 minutes. When done, unmold and place on a platter. You can garnish with any fresh or steamed vegetables.

Baked Rum Bananas

This is one of my easiest and favorite concoctions—but it was so easy that for a long time I resisted making it for my guests, figuring they deserved a more complicated and "sophisticated" dessert. Wrong! It is always a hit, and it's one of those desserts that can accommodate a last-minute guest—just add another banana.

>   8 bananas, not too ripe
>   1 teaspoon unsalted margarine, for greasing baking
>   dish
>   ½ cup brown sugar
>   ½ cup rum
>   1 teaspoon ground cinnamon
>   ½ teaspoon ground cloves
>   Pinch nutmeg
>   ½ cup lemon juice
>   ½ cup toasted slivered almonds

Preheat oven to 350°.

Slice the bananas horizontally and place them, cut side down, in one layer in a large glass baking dish which has been lightly greased. Mix all the other ingredients, except the almonds, in a bowl and pour over the bananas.

Bake for 15–20 minutes. When done, put one half of a banana slice on each dessert plate, pour some hot sauce over each, and top with the almonds. Serve immediately, while still hot. SERVES 16 (Add one whole banana for each additional person; you don't have to prepare any more sauce until you make over 14 bananas.)

EATING OUT

It's pretty easy to be "good" when you entertain at home, isn't it? After all, *you* control what you make, you decide on which foods you will serve, you make the meals both nutritious and delicious—no problem! But eating out is something else entirely. How can you go to a restaurant and read a menu full of "forbidden foods" and still expect to be served foods that are on our nutritious list? How can you dine at a friend's house and not eat the sour cream and chives, the rare steak dripping with fat, the creamed-chocolate cake that the hostess baked with her own little hands?

Whether you eat out at a restaurant or at a friend's home, you are presented with a "fait accompli"—here is dinner, and you will eat it and you will like it! Right? Well, maybe. It's actually easier to stay on the Diet to Lose and the Diet for Life than you think. All you have to do is remember a few things.

Have Fun!

First—eating out is fun. Much as we may like our own cooking, much as we may enjoy entertaining at home, it is fun to visit friends at their homes, or to go out on the town to a party or to a dinner at a restaurant.

As you already know, I love to entertain at home, but I also treasure those moments spent at friends' homes, sharing great company and wonderful food. And I relish visiting different restaurants, enjoying the various decors, sampling foods on intriguing menus, and generally having a grand time.

So make up your mind that your first priority is to have a great time—you'll take care of the food question later.

Be Flexible

Nothing on the Diet to Lose or on the Diet for Life is cast in stone. There is always an alternative, a solution or if worse comes to worst, you'll eat a little of the steak and tomorrow you'll feast on salad. Eating out should not be a hassle or an insurmountable problem. If you become that concerned with what you are going to eat, you'll take all the joy out of going out and you'll wish you had just stayed home. Forget this attitude! Use the tools I will give you to handle the food situation in the best possible way, and then sit back and have the time of your life.

Don't Be Intimidated!

Easier said than done? I know. I too have come across the waiter who, when asked if he can bring your salad with the dressing on the side, replies quite arrogantly, "Madam, we make no changes!" (I also ran into one who looked at me with great disgust when I asked for yogurt instead of sour cream and chives for my baked potato. Bringing himself up to his very greatest height, he replied, "You won't like it," and brought me the largest dish of sour cream and chives I have ever seen!)

Don't be intimidated by such types. I have since learned never to *ask* a waiter for his opinion, but to say politely with a smile (always with a smile), "I'd like my dressing on the side, please" instead of "Can I have . . . ," or "I'd appreciate your leaving the sauce on the side" instead of "Would you mind . . . ." And don't apologize for asking for what you want: "I'm really sorry to bother you, but do you think that it might be possible for you, if you have a minute, to bring me the dressing on the side?" is guaranteed to get you a big, fat "No!"

A positive attitude almost always works. Invert your question into a simple request and you are likely to be met with respect and a quick "Yes, Madam." Start with the assumption that you deserve to get what you want. Remember, restaurants are there to serve you—you are the customer, and the customer *is* always right!

These three basic principles—have fun, be flexible, and don't be intimidated—will carry you far. There are some additional ways of dealing with situations that can arise when any of us who are careful about the foods we eat decide to eat out.

Eating at Friends' Homes

Although it is easier to diet at the home of someone you know, it does present some problems of its own. Because we care about our friends, we are often reluctant to put them to any extra trouble. Thus when confronted by a homecooked meal we would not dream of eating at home, we are often "self-intimidated" into eating it anyway.

There is a better way—it's called being "carefully honest," and it goes like this:

1. When you are invited to a friend's home, if the subject of food comes up, gently and easily mention to your host that you are watching what you eat. Don't make a big deal out of this—remember that eating on any of the *Diet Principal* programs means you have some flexibility in what you can and what you will want to eat. Don't dictate a list of the forbidden foods to your host—this will not make her happy, nor will you ever be invited over again. A simple comment like the following works best: "I've been eating lightly lately, so don't worry about what to make for me—the simpler, the better."

2. When you talk to your hostess before the party, see if you can find out what's going to be on the menu. This doesn't mean an inquisition ("I'd like to know what you are serving, because I don't eat most foods and to avoid a problem I'd like to be prepared in case I have to bring my own dinner."). This kind of conversation is unnecessary. A simple "What are you making for dinner?" will do. Knowing what will be served will better prepare you. If the dinner is heavy in fatty foods and sauces that are going to cause havoc in your diet, you'll be able to eat lightly before you go to the party and will eat less once you are there.

3. When you arrive and see a buffet full of salami, olives, peppers and anchovies in olive oil, cheeses galore, and rare roast beef surrounded by potato salad made with mayonnaise, don't panic. Salvage as much of the fresh food as possible, and if that's easier said than done, just take a little bit of the least objectionable foods you can find—crackers, a little dip, fruit, etc.

4. When you are confronted with a sit-down dinner and the food is too rich for you, don't announce it to those present. Quietly taste a little bit of everything so as not to insult your host. (Actually, that's a well-known trick of food critics—you taste a bit of everything, but you never finish anything so you minimize your weight gain.) If you are served a salad, ask for a second helping, and eat the bread (leave out the butter). That way you will fill yourself up and can leave out some of the more objectionable foods—red meats, fatty sauces, etc.

5. If you find out that one of the dishes is a host's home-made specialty, eat it. Even if it's full of fat, it won't hurt you to eat it once and it will make her feel terrific. This is not a license to go crazy every night of the week—always keep in mind that cheating only leads to more fat on your thighs and in your arteries. But for an occasional party remember that, whatever you eat, it's only one meal, and you can always compensate tomorrow by eating better and less.

Always keep this fundamental principle in mind—have a good time, but not at the expense of your health. Eat and drink moderately, the latter particularly if you are planning to drive home.

Eating Out in a Restaurant

Once you have made up your mind to have fun, to be flexible, and not to be intimidated, you are ready to enjoy eating at a restaurant while on a diet. And I mean enjoy—eating out while dieting need not be a chore, or a nutritional nightmare. Actually, it will be fun. All you need to know are the following principles:

1. Let's start with the easy part. Because of the renewed interest in nutrition on the part of both the public and restaurant owners, many restaurants are now offering "light" menus and/or dishes that contain more nutritious food and less fat. Even some fast food places, such as McDonald's and Wendy's, are offering salads and "diet specials" which can fit your diet beautifully. In general it is easier now to eat out than it was even a couple of years ago.

But along with "progress" come some warnings. Many diet specials are not good for you. Witness a typical menu at an ordinary hangout for lunch—the diet special includes ground sirloin, cottage cheese, and canned fruit in syrup. On that diet you can consume over 700 calories (and digest a lot of fat and sodium) in one fell swoop!

Thus, sometimes it is better to rely on your own knowledge about what food is good for you. In Chapter 2 you learned what's in what you eat, and you now have at least a rudimentary knowledge of good nutrition. You really are the best person to choose what to eat at a time like this. So ignore "diet" dishes that you know contain foods you don't want, and select your own.

2. Some dishes have "stay away from me" written all over them. Deep-fried shrimp or tortilla chips, cream soups, melted cheese sandwiches (which have been fried in oil) are the obvious. If a menu is chock full of these "goodies," pick out something you can eat, like a salad or a baked potato, and order two. This will ensure that you get a nutritious lunch without going hungry.

3. As I said above, always feel free to ask for the food to be prepared the way you like it. If fish is on the menu, unless it is prepared way in advance (in which case you may want to reconsider eating there) it is simple to have the chef merely broil the fish and leave off the cream sauce. The same goes for chicken or turkey. This is especially important on the Diet to Lose because you really can't afford to eat that cream or deep-fried food. So don't be afraid to ask!

4. When you reach for the butter knife, first ask whether those little yellow pats of fat are butter or margarine, then spread the bread accordingly. I prefer not to use either—you don't need the extra fat and the bread tastes just fine without it.

5. One night while I was eating at a restaurant in Dallas, I noticed a woman at the next table reading a little booklet while she was preparing to order her meal. When she got up to go to the ladies' room, I discreetly followed her. She thought I wanted to mug her, but what I wanted to know was what she had been reading. It turned out she carried with her a tiny booklet published by the American Heart Association containing information and tips on eating out. (For your free copy, write the American Heart Association National Center, 7320 Greenville Avenue, Dallas, Texas 75231.) Here are some invaluable tips on reading menus that I learned from this booklet:

- Learn which terms and phrases telegraph low-fat preparation. Look for:

steamed	garden fresh
in its own juice	broiled, roasted, poached

- Be aware that some low-fat, low-cholesterol preparations are high in sodium. Watch out for foods that are:

pickled	in a tomato base
smoked	in cocktail sauce
in broth	

- Menu descriptions that warn of saturated fat and cholesterol preparation may also indicate high sodium. Avoid foods that are:

buttery or buttered	braised
in its own gravy	creamed, or in cream sauce
sautéed	hollandaise
fried	marinated in oil
panfried	basted
crispy	casserole

6. Before going out to dinner, have a snack at home. Snacking will take the edge off your appetite and will fill you up sufficiently so that you won't be starving when you arrive. Just as I suggest you eat before you go food shopping in the supermarket (you're less likely to buy foods you don't need, and more likely to buy less of everything), so it is a good idea to eat a little before you go out to dinner. In this way you will order less, and eat more carefully.

7. After being on the Diet to Lose and the Diet for Life for a while, you will automatically know how much of each food you can safely and nutritiously have at one sitting. You will need this knowledge because at most restaurants, bigger is better. Quantity, not necessarily quality, is the rule most restaurants seem to live by.

The good news is that it will be second nature to you to know when a dish contains enough nutritious food and when it has too much of everything in it. Don't bring along a scale; don't worry about the portions you are served. Merely eat as much as you know will be good for you. And don't overdo— it is so tempting to want to clean your plate at a restaurant! But forget it—let the dishwashers clean it.

8. Just because you are in a restaurant doesn't mean you can forget some basics, like drinking iced tea before or after your meal. The same benefits apply here as they did at home.

9. If your dinner or lunch out is a business affair, you may be under more pressure and thus be more self-conscious than usual. But as long as you don't make your dietary habits an issue, you can still stick to your diet plan. Just order whatever you would have, without making a point of what you are eating. And try choosing the restaurant, if you can, because going to a place with which you are familiar or where you are known may make things easier.

Eating on an Airplane

There are two things that are always true about an airplane: one, that it will fly in the air, and two, that the food will be—now how can I be tactful—not great, and fattening. But you don't have to be a prisoner of the meals served on a flight.

Anyone can call the airline a day or so before a flight and order a so-called "special" meal. You don't have to be a vegetarian to order the "vegetarian special," which is really a salad, a fruit plate, or steamed vegetables, all of which tend to be fresher, better-tasting, and more nutritious than those ordinary meals. You don't have to eat those sausages and cheese, the little ham snacks, or the salted peanuts. If you like to snack, take along a fruit or a package of unsalted potato chips, almonds, or dried apricots. Thinking ahead can make your flight much more pleasurable and less of a nutritional nightmare.

An added note: the air pressure in the cabin of an airplane will make your skin dry and may also play havoc with your digestive system. Take along a package of Tums (this will also take care of your calcium intake), and be sure to drink a lot of water during the flight. You can also ask for our old favorite, iced tea—not out of a can, but fresh. The stewardess will be delighted to make you some.

Always remember that eating out should be a pleasure. Whether you are eating at a restaurant or at a friend's home, the point is to have a good time without compromising your eating habits too much. Moderation and balance, together with these principles, will make for a great time out wherever you are.

EPILOGUE

Now go to it. You have all the tools that you will need right at your fingertips. You understand why you eat too much, and how to take control of your eating habits so that you can establish a new way of eating intelligently and healthfully. You know how your body works and what the foods, both beneficial and harmful, do to your body. You have the Diet to Lose and the Diet for Life, both of which will ensure that you never again need to search for another way to lose weight. You have the recipes so that you can easily and deliciously prepare food for your own family and your friends. And most of all, you have the Diet Principles, which will always help you stick to your beliefs, remind you to take care of yourself, and give you the tools with which you will successfully remain healthy and beautiful for the rest of your life.

It's up to you. You can do it, so go for it—today!

INDEX